SEE?

LIVING BLIND IN A
SIGHTED WORLD

By Sandra Fortier

Edited by Nancy LaFever

Printed in the United States of America
Published by Braughler Books LLC., Springboro, Ohio

First printing, 2021

ISBN: 978-1-970063-82-0

Library of Congress Control Number: 2021910700

Ordering information: Special discounts are available on quantity purchases by bookstores, corporations, associations, and others. For details, contact the publisher at:

sales@braughlerbooks.com

or at 937-58-BOOKS

For questions or comments about this book, please write to:

info@braughlerbooks.com

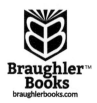

Braughler™
Books
braughlerbooks.com

Table of Contents

ACKNOWLEDGEMENTS

GOD MADE THIS ALL POSSIBLE!

In 2009, Mr. Roderick Magoon, a former eighth-grade science teacher at Ella White School, planted the seeds for this book including the title See? as an attention grabber in its irony. He instilled self-confidence, love of learning, yet respect for boundaries.

God also brought me to Mrs. Lori Mansell-Solinski, Prime Life Enrichment Follies organizer, and her daughter, Julie Osborne. They were key pivotal players in discovering Braughler Books LLC and Nancy LaFever, editor, who realized this dream of sharing my story with others.

Don't forget other supporting characters in this cast: A. D. Ruedemann, a former ophthalmologist, and my parents, Joseph and Virginia Fortier. Accolades to my sister and brother-in-law, Nancy and John Fezzey, other teachers, choral directors, clergy, countless friends, and neighbors who encouraged me to live a normal life despite limited vision.

I also extend special appreciation to the National Federation of the Blind Writers' Division; Pam Bortz, Hadley Institute for the Blind English Composition instructor; and Steve Tearman, Indiana Oasis Instructor.

Employment as a word processing assistant at the Michigan Commission for the Blind Training Center introduced me to life-enhancing adaptive technology. Center staff mentoring and friendship over the years have enriched my life.

INTRODUCTION

"It's a girl!" announced my debut into the world followed by Dr. Wienczewski's astonished, "Another one! Mrs. Fortier, you have twins!" heralding Nancy's surprising arrival.

Inwardly, Mother must have reacted with both joy and misgivings. "How am I going to take care of two babies let alone one?" I can also imagine her face etched with worry and her body drenched with perspiration and writhing in pain before collapsing into complete exhaustion. I cannot fathom her carrying and delivering twins from a 5-foot, 100-pound body.

In contrast, Dad physically presented himself with a ruggedly handsome face framed by thick, wavy, black hair and a bright, welcoming smile crinkling the corners of his hazel eyes. His strong arms and broad shoulders flanked a stocky 5' 8" build. Growing up on a farm and playing baseball for the Indian Reserve team developed this physique. Despite his hardiness, he characterized the young father-to-be nervously pacing in the hospital waiting room.

Finally hearing the news that he had twin daughters, Dad immediately bought another carton of cigarettes to pass around at Besser Manufacturing Company where he then worked as a crane operator. During the celebration at work the following week, his friends cheered, "Way to go, Joe!" while thumping him on the back.

Nancy and I grew up in Alpena, located in the northern part of the Lower Peninsula within the mitten-shaped state of Michigan. Though we have always joked about the pungent odor Abitibi Paper Mill spewed and the "cement plant specials," cars corroded by Huron Portland cement dust, Alpena was an ideal place in which to grow up during the 1950s, because it was unscathed by the present crime scourge. Therefore, I link it to happy, early childhood memories. In one, Dad pushed the sleigh in which my sister and I sat bundled up in navy blue snowsuits, mittens, and hats with ear flaps that tied under the chin. Others include summer evenings when we sipped root beer from frosty mugs or rode with the car windows open to keep cool while listening to Ernie Harwell announce the Detroit Tiger baseball games. How could we ever forget the drive-in movies and band concerts, our inability to refrain from peeking as Mom hid Easter baskets in the vestibule, and laughter while coloring Easter eggs representing popular movie stars, such as Doris Day, Eartha Kitt, and Jayne Mansfield? Later chapters will deal with other childhood memories.

Nancy and I were raised in a loving atmosphere in which most relatives, teachers, neighbors, and adult friends instilled within us positive attitudes, a strong work ethic, and the value of higher education. Though twins, Nancy and I both developed into distinctly different personalities, she as a witty extrovert and I, a subtly humored introvert.

Fast forward to an autumn Sunday in 1973 when I was 24 years old. At a Kalamazoo, Michigan church, another choir member remarked following our singing the recessional hymn, "Too bad you have to look so close at your hymnal. Were you born that way? Didn't anybody do something about that?" I explained, "I have limited vision due to premature birth; however, I believe that things happen for a reason. Perhaps God gave me enough vision to appreciate the beauty but also to protect me against seeing and only dwelling on the vices that the world contains." This book will describe a fulfilling life due to God's grace in guiding me through the challenges of blindness.

CHAPTER 1: THROUGH MY LENS

My twin sister, Nancy, and I were born prematurely, only seven-month babies. Being 2 lbs. 7 oz. guaranteed me a two-month incubator hospital stay.

About a year later, Mother noticed when I was reaching for toys and utensils, I looked away from them instead of directly at them. My eyes continually rolled in my head so that she could only see the whites. Alarmed, Mother took me to Dr. Kessler, my pediatrician, for examination. He advised, "If Sandy were my daughter, I'd take her to the University of Michigan in Ann Arbor or to Dr. A. D. Ruedemann in Detroit." Being familiar with Detroit, having worked there from 1942 until 1947 at Western Union and then as a secretary at Square D, Mother chose Dr. Ruedemann.

I do not remember much about this visit except gazing in awe out his waiting room window at what appeared to be toy cars, trucks, and buses zooming along a narrow thoroughfare like a toy train on a track.

During the examination, Dr. Ruedemann handed me a paper cup filled with water. Being so thirsty, did I ever grab it and gulp the water! Then, I didn't realize that he was really assessing eye/hand coordination. After observing this and my walking, to Mother's relief as she told me in later years, he declared, "I wish many other young parents did the same for their children as you did for Sandy by bringing her in. That child is nearsighted, not totally blind. She has a keen mind. See that she gets all the education that she can. In school she will need to sit in the front seat close to the blackboard and be teacher's pet."

Dr. Ruedemann diagnosed me with myopia, meaning nearsightedness, and retinopathy at prematurity, a disease in which too much oxygen in the incubator causes an abnormal growth of blood vessels from the retina into the back of the eye, leakage, and retinal scarring. He added that I would eventually outgrow the nystagmus which is involuntary jerking of the eyes and reassured Mother that my vision would either remain stable or improve.

Like wavy funhouse mirrors, limited vision distorts perceptions of people and objects. At a very tender age, for instance, I wondered why a pink-and-white polka dot dress seemed light pink to me; whereas another person saw polka dots at a distance as well as nearby. Flowered wallpaper of hydrangeas, daisies, and roses on blue or green background, for instance, seen from a distance resembled colored blobs against a green or sky-blue construction paper backdrop. Naturally, I wanted to go close to that woman to see if the dress was polka-dotted or to the wall to discover what the blobs really were.

Besides the frustration of being unable to see something up close, poor vision spawned early childhood terrors I eventually outgrew by Mother's tough love approach in dealing with them and improved vision. Though I enjoyed receiving Halloween candy, that was where the fun began for Nancy–and ended for me. Aunt Vina's Spooktacular mazy gauntlet of ghosts, skeletons, witches, and goblins hanging on every wall and in every corner tickled me as I ran through it, terrifying me until I became old enough to realize that they were artificial. As an additional scary prop, Bill, a cousin six years older than me, often sneaked up behind me, hollering, "Boo! The bogeyman will get you!"

Stemming from a three-year-old's imagination and poor vision, other things frightened me besides Bill's impersonation of the bogeyman and Aunt Vina's Halloween decorations. Associating a vehicle's huge glaring headlights, which I could only see at a distance and the sound of its air brakes with the demonic eyes and hissing of fire-breathing dragons vividly portrayed in fairy tales, for instance, I was extremely afraid of trucks and buses as I crossed Detroit's Woodward Avenue from our hotel to the David Whitney Building which housed Dr. Ruedemann's office. "Don't be frightened!" pleaded Mother. "These aren't dragons going to hurt you. They're only trucks and buses stopping to let us cross. Hurry up!"

4

I also cowered and screamed whenever Mother wore a red ski jacket including a red hood trimmed with white fur, because she appeared like a fox to me at a distance. To help me overcome this fear, she made me wear the jacket several times, reassuring, "See, it's nothing to be afraid of."

Located around M-32 in Alpena and owned by Percy Clemmons, a close friend of Aunt Vina's and our families, my other nemesis as a toddler was a log-cabin camp, which could have portrayed a scene for a spine-chilling play or movie. Reaching the camp necessitated climbing mud steps which faced a secondary road overrun with brambles and massive trees darkening the forest even on sunny days. This road wound many miles from the main road. As if enveloped in a ghostly silence, I could hear no sounds of people or animals around the camp.

Inside the camp, acrid cigarette smoke curled in eerie hazy halos around kerosene lamps. Then I recoiled and screamed at what I thought was a bear lying on a couch from a distance. After Mother led me to the couch and told me to feel it while she explained, "It's only a couch of black bearskins," I sat on it.

My present visual acuity of 20/200 means that what most people can see at 200 feet, I can only see at 20. Besides lacking central vision, I am therefore declared legally blind. Yet, to Mother's and Dr. Ruedemann's amazement, I could distinguish colors even at an early age. Having difficulty detecting facial expressions and body language, I rely solely on voices to recognize people.

Unable to see detail at a distance, even today, I still am extremely frustrated with art and museum exhibits that are roped off or encased in glass, because I rely on the sense of touch to enhance what I see. Lacking depth perception, I find escalators and circular staircases very deceiving, as well as contrasting colors of carpeting or tile emerging as steps to me even though the floor is flat.

As another illustration of visual distortion, imagine a vase on a table at a distance with the table the same color as brown wainscoting. I can only see the dark backdrop and flowers as splotchy colors suspended in midair. With a lighter backdrop, I can see a square representing the two legs of the table and the flowers suspended in midair.

I use a white cane for identification and detecting drop-offs, curbs, bumps on sidewalks, climbing steps, and crossing streets while traveling outdoors or in unfamiliar places indoors.

My reminiscing with Mother about this aspect of my life from 1951 to 1954 echoes Dr. Ruedemann's praises of her and illustrates the magnitude of prayer.

"Mom, how did you ride that Greyhound bus to and from Detroit and stay alone with me in strange hotel rooms every three months we visited Dr. Ruedemann? Think back to waiting for restrooms until we stopped at diners!"

"Well, Sandy, I was young and gutsier than I am now."

Continuing, Mother sobbed, "I loved you so much! Taking you to the best eye doctor, I hoped that you'd see well enough to go to school and play like other children."

"What alternative did I have? I didn't drive then, and Dad had to work. Later when your vision improved to where you were only required to see Dr. Ruedemann once every two years, Dad drove us to Detroit during his vacation time when we either stayed with Aunt Florence or in motels." Aunt Florence, Dad's sister, lived a block near the Shrine of the Little Flower in Royal Oak, Michigan, a suburb of Detroit.

"Do you remember how we prayed to Mary and the baby Jesus when Aunt Florence took us to the Shrine of the Little Flower?"

"Yes, Mom. The shrine was a dark, though a serene place where I always prayed as if I were nestled in His loving adult arms, 'Jesus, please make my eyes good.' To me, candles and statues appeared in grottos on the walls. The pews were positioned like seats inside a theater in the round."

Until I read a brochure on the Shrine of the Little Flower in Royal Oak, I would have never known that the "candles and statues in grottos" were stained-glass windows and lanterns suspended from the ceiling. Nor would I have seen the solid, pure white marble altar located in the center of the church to illustrate one's faith centered on the sacrifice of the mass being celebrated. Two peacocks drinking from a fountain in front of the altar symbolized everlasting life, and the wounded and victorious lamb on the opposite side of the altar represented the Risen Christ. Wheat and grapes on the corners of the altar symbolized the Holy Eucharist. In contrast, from my standpoint, blotches of color were meaningless to me. Only seeing the church interior at a distance, but not having read this information, how I would have missed its awesome splendor!

Thanks to Mother's vigilance, our prayer power, and Dr. Ruedemann's exemplary care, my vision finally improved to 20/200 as it has been for most of my adult life. Comparing this to 20/20 vision, most people would merely regard it as a pebble alongside a rock. To Mother and Dad, however, it was a miracle.

CHAPTER 2: LAUNCHING INTO LIFE

Arriving home from the hospital in April 1949 after spending two months in the incubator, I lived with my family in an upstairs apartment on 306 Lockwood Street. I only vaguely recall bathing in a high bathtub on legs. There was a hole reminding me of a navel in the wall behind the tub.

When Nancy and I were two years old, our family moved to 123 West Blair, a home located on the corner of Third and Blair. For several years, it was gray cement block with a vestibule in front and a cellar in back. Later, a front porch with an overhang and columns replaced the vestibule. I remember more clearly the house re-painted brown with white trim and the cellar torn down and remodeled into a garage.

As toddlers, Nancy and I happily played in the backyard but hated the fence that protected us from heavy traffic. We spent many hours pretending we were making cookies with the sugar sand in our red wooden sandbox. This abruptly ended when one of the neighborhood children used the sandbox as a toilet.

How we especially enjoyed splashing in our kiddie pool on summer days! It was a round mint green plastic pool with a white Mickey Mouse on the bottom. During the winter, the wooden cellar doors made an ideal slide until Dad, concerned about our safety, curtailed that activity.

My parents never regarded me as handicapped or tolerated laziness. "Either help around the house or get a job," they urged. While working full time at Besser Manufacturing Company and part-time as a licensed electrician, Dad expected Nancy and me to pull our weight. Mother, the quintessential homemaker, ran our household as a captain runs a tight ship. Nancy and I washed dishes, cleaned our rooms, ironed, mowed, and trimmed grass, washed garage windows, swept sidewalks, and shoveled snow. Using techniques of repetitive movement and feeling for dirt, Mother taught me household tasks of sweeping, dusting, and vacuuming.

Through an ulterior motive of avoiding bending within such a narrow space, one day, I gave the grass between the fence and the garage a brush cut with the trimmer. Seeing what I had done and kicking the ground, Mother scolded, "My God! What possessed you?"

"Mom," I protested. "I couldn't see well enough to tell."

"You know better than that! Anything to get out of work! But I'm not letting you off that easy. We're going to buy and plant new grass seed to fill in this space. Don't you ever use poor vision as an excuse again!" Indeed, I learned my lesson!

Since my difficulty in cracking eggs nearly drove Mother crazy with exasperation, I did not cook or bake much until I had my own apartment. Through trial and error, I eventually mastered this technique. Then, I would have enjoyed baking more, however, if I had been taught to crack eggs through repetitive motion, instead of by observation, or if I had the presently marketed devices combining the processes of cracking, separating, and scrambling eggs.

Thus, doubting myself as ever becoming the most accomplished cook and gracious hostess as she was, I both admired and envied Mother. She prepared meals for our family and many guests. Mother's kitchen also hummed while she created hors d'oeuvres for parties she hosted and goodies for school parties and church bake sales. Mouth-watering aromas of bacon and eggs, sausage, pot roasts, breaded chicken and pork chops, creamed turkey, chop suey, meatballs, cream puffs, various cakes, and pies pervaded the whole house. Generally more outgoing than I and interested in people, my parents successfully drew out the most bashful at parties they hosted, encouraging guests to "eat slowly and eat lots" and to help themselves to open-bar beverages. Though Mother reassured me that with practice I would learn how to cook and entertain as well as she did, I regarded her as a tough act to follow.

I cherish other fond Christmas memories, especially a childhood fantasy in which Nancy and I eagerly anticipated Santa's appearance through the fireplace, though cardboard, after his climbing down the chimney. How we enjoyed singing Christmas carols with Uncle Leonard, one of mother's brothers who had a beautiful singing voice, and Midnight Mass where I completely immersed myself in the music, or visiting Aunt Vina's house, which on a small-scale replicated Bronner's Christmas Store in Frankenmuth, Michigan. Her meals, especially her cheesecake made with Holland Rusk and cottage cheese, were generally delicious except for her seashell macaroni and pineapple salad which Nancy and I disliked but ate to be polite. Of course, we devoured Dad's relatives' homemade cookies and traditional French meat pies or *tourtières* with Mother's being the best. Though reaching the saturation point by New Year's Day after eating so many meat pies, again our palates craved them soon as the holidays rolled around the following year!

Our Sunday drives and summer vacations comprised a patchwork quilt of many places and interesting experiences. We zigzagged through a labyrinth of country roads along Hubbard, Long, and Grand Lakes, and Presque Isle and drove around Dad's cedar-shingled boyhood home where he grew up with eight other siblings. Although its windows were boarded up, its front door was unlocked. So, we did explore Bunker School, a two-room schoolhouse that Dad attended as a child on Indian Reserve Road then located in Wilson Township near Alpena, Michigan. We attended many drive-in movies, Alpena Fourth of July parades, spectacular fireworks displays, band concerts, Traverse City cherry and Posen potato festivals.

I always looked forward to the tasty wiener and marshmallow roasts behind the Huron Portland Cement Plant with Aunt Vina, my cousins Lillian, Jeannie, and Bill. Riding under the gate that looked like a viaduct, I imagined entering the moat of a castle. Mesmerized by the bonfire, I felt as if I were relaxing in front of a cozy fireplace in someone's living room.

Heedless of damp, cold, rainy weather, we also often picnicked together around Harrisville Park on Memorial Day holiday weekends when Dad treated us to homemade ice cream, cranking the ice cream maker with rock salt. Never hardening, the ice cream tasted like a rich French vanilla milkshake.

Besides summer vacations and picnics, church attendance and activities have always played a vital role in our family life. When St. John the Baptist Catholic Church was built on Frederick Street in Alpena, Dad eagerly volunteered his time as an electrician, and Mother served on umpteen church committees involving dinners, bake sales, and rummage sales. She even assigned Nancy and me the job of making price tags for rummage sales, though I must admit that sorting through the clothes as browsers in vintage clothing stores took higher priority over making the price tags.

Mother and Dad assumed that any child, regardless of disability, should try new things, even though the outcome might not always be successful. An avid ice skater while in high school and working in Detroit, Mother suggested skating as one possible fun-filled family activity. Each Sunday afternoon, we alternated between the rinks at Mich-E-Ke-Wis Park on US 23 South and McRae Park on Merchant Street across the river. Absolute purgatory!

Afraid of falling, I wobbled on skates instead of gliding across the ice with the ease and gracefulness of Peggy Fleming. Mother's coaxing, "You have to fall to learn," backfired in her intent to motivate me since it increased my fear of falling. Children's taunts, "Do you have polio?" embarrassed me. To my relief, Mother eventually discontinued ice skating.

Watching Nancy as a spunky eight-year-old whizzing around our block on a neighbor's bicycle that she had learned to ride, I also wanted a bicycle. Recalling my refusal to ride my tricycle which appeared too high for me, Mother and Dad initially hesitated to buy me a bike. Finally relenting after I proved my readiness to ride one, Mother and Dad bought Nancy and me Schwinn bicycles for our ninth birthday.

Since mine had training wheels, I confidently rode it until the screws on the training wheels loosened and fell off. My parents did not recommend training wheels after that because I relied on them too much. Throughout that entire summer, Dad took me to the Ella

White School playground where I practiced riding my two-wheeler, first getting my balance there. I did have more trouble gaining balance while riding on the sidewalk which appeared so narrow compared to the playground, but I persevered. Finally, I rode the bike without falling! Now I could accompany Nancy on errands and excursions. We went around town to beaches, parks, small boat harbor, historical buildings, and the Alpena Public Library where on hot summer days Nancy and I searched for books in its dark, comfortingly cool, and quiet atmosphere.

The next summer, Mother signed Nancy and me up for bowling at the Thunder Bowl on US 23 South and swimming lessons at Bayview Park on State Street. Mrs. Decker, the swimming instructor, taught me by moving my arms and legs required for the various strokes, such as the crawl, the dog paddle, and the breaststroke, which I easily learned. Bowling was a different story. Although Mother and I informed the bowling instructor about my limited vision, she demonstrated the approach five alleys away from me. Therefore, I could not imitate her movements of synchronizing the steps–one, two, three, slide–with throwing the ball. Believing that I was too old to walk to the foul line, bend over, and throw the ball, Dad taught me the approach. I mastered it once he directed me to feel his movements while he bowled and then guided me through each step after he positioned me in the correct stance.

Replacing Mrs. Decker, our former swimming teacher, the following year, Mr. Gillespie offered children swimming lessons in the river by the Alpena County Fairgrounds, because it was deeper than Bayview Park and Mich-E-Ke-Wis beaches, though it teemed with slime, muck, algae, and drop-offs. Miraculously, we did not drown and contract tetanus or anything else such as H1N1 virus and Lyme disease. Rain or shine, Mr. Gillespie reviewed strokes and emphasized endurance. Passing advanced beginners required all the energy and the courage that I could muster to swim the required length of the river and to dive from the boat into the water.

Unlike those swimming lessons, I enjoyed the Alpena County Fair. The carousel calliope greeted fair-goers with a waltz or a march. Horses' hooves pounded on the racetrack. Aromas of popcorn, cotton candy, corn dogs, burgers, fries, onion rings, and elephant ears wafted from various concession stands. Passing by the Adults Only tents, I wondered what forbidden secrets they concealed. I rode the Tilt-A-Whirl, Ferris Wheel, Scrambler, and Bumper Cars with Dad guiding the steering wheel.

One day he suggested, "Sandy, here's a real dare-devil ride for you, the Loop O Plane! How would you like that?" It consisted of two Dutch shoes suspended from a rotating wheel, revolving upside down. I could hardly wait!

"Now here we go!" Dad crowed. Though intended to be fun, the ride somersaulted me into a death-defying feat because the operator failed to strap me securely into the seat. This left me flopping inside, clinging to the bar. What would I do? Would I fall out? I would not admit I was scared. Thank God, I was not injured!

This was one of many life's Loop O Planes I rode.

CHAPTER 3: A DILEMMA

Dr. Ruedemann and my parents advocated main-streaming visually impaired children in the public schools 30 years ahead of their time, while most blind children attended residential schools. Thus, Mother and Dad reasoned, "Why shouldn't Sandy begin attending regular elementary school classes, since she will compete with sighted adults eventually when she attends college or seeks employment?"

I believe that my poor eyesight brought our whole family closer to God in our increasing reliance upon Him. Before I entered school, for instance, a family friend suggested that we attend Mother of Perpetual Help novenas held at St. Anne's Catholic Church on 817 Sable Street. I always looked forward to these novenas in this cathedral-style church where reflections from stained glass windows bounced on the walls during sunny evenings like reflections through prisms hanging from a chandelier. Depicting Jesus' life, distant images within these windows, however, appeared blurry to me. The domed ceiling was painted white with apple-red blobs which Mother informed me were crosses symbolizing Jesus Christ's Precious Blood shed for our sins. The side and back walls were painted dusty pink, and the wall behind the altar and its dome were painted light blue. How I wish a magical hoist could have lifted me up so I could see the ceilings and columns in more detail! I furtively glanced around the cathedral to avoid Mother's eagle eye and her ensuing nudges also given when I rocked to the liturgical music. Mother worried about blindisms, which are annoying behaviors including rocking or eye pressing that blind children exhibit to provide stimulation. Listening to the ethereal-sounding choir singing Latin responses and hymns, I thought I caught a glimpse of heaven. From the time I started kindergarten until I graduated from high school, my family and I prayerfully attended those novenas, hoping this would assist me in adjusting to regular classes.

I did not realize how treacherous this journey through public school would be when I joyfully anticipated that first day of kindergarten. As soon as Mother left me in the classroom, I darted toward the boys' corner, playing with a shiny new red truck. As police officers catch speeders on their radar, Mrs. Stone then swooped down, yanked the truck away from me, and ordered me to play in the girls' corner. "You know girls play with dolls, not with trucks!" On the other hand, my parents knew that I detested dolls. Give me a toy typewriter, piano, cash register, truck, or car to play with, and I was in seventh heaven.

Undaunted, I undid a roll of Scotch tape, held it up to my eyes, wondering why the tape was transparent and tried to rewind it in the spool. I also sharpened crayons in the pencil sharpener. Besides touching the projector, I hovered around Mrs. Stone, watching her type to see how a typewriter operated. Naturally, this would annoy anyone, but as a five-year-old child, I did not understand why her patience wore thin by my countless antics. Being curious, I was also extremely frustrated by my inability to ask questions regarding the operation of these machines.

I also had difficulty conforming to instructions, "It's cleanup time!" or "Nap time!" and with drawing and coloring inside the lines. After Mrs. Stone sent me home with a note, that weekend my parents bought me a pencil sharpener and showed me its correct usage. To grasp the concept of geometric figures and coloring within the lines, I also practiced drawing lines, circles, squares, and triangles on the chalkboard in my bedroom and coloring in coloring books.

Still doubting my ability to function in a regular class, Mrs. Stone recommended that my parents investigate the Michigan School for the Blind as alternative education for me. This they did reluctantly, however, knowing they would face the formidable challenge of relocating home, family, and job to Lansing, Michigan.

Waiting to visit MSB seemed like an eternity to me, because I longed for a teacher who would allow me to do what I wanted. When the day finally arrived, I was gleeful but oblivious to my parents' anxieties regarding my adjustment to the new school, our possible relocation to Lansing, and transportation to and from Lansing every weekend if a job opening did not materialize for Dad at the Lansing Besser Company branch.

During the trip to Lansing, I hopped from the front seat into the back and climbed on top of the seat to look out the window at passing cars, signs, people, and animals that captured my interest. No wonder Mom and Dad were dog-tired when we arrived there!

Entering the school the next morning, I could hardly contain myself! As I ran from one classroom to another, my parents could not keep up with me. Finally, Dad clamped a viselike grip on my arm.

Soon the director introduced me to Mrs. Keifer, the kindergarten teacher who kept me in her charge for the whole day while my parents toured the school with him. The room was octagonal shaped with a white piano on which Mrs. Keifer played children's songs. This I thoroughly enjoyed, naturally loving music and singing. Then playtime arrived—and bedlam broke loose! Some children scurried to build block towers. Others played house. Those with more vision played hide-and-seek. I was heading toward the sandbox when clunk! Something like a mallet crashed against the back of my head, and did it sting! Unable to consider that the children could not see me, I did not get out of their way. Despite all this, I really wanted to stay.

How dismayed my parents felt at the sight awaiting them as the tour progressed! They later informed me that the dormitory room shown to them was painted a drab institutional blue and installed with a bare tile floor to prevent tripping over rugs. Beds were dark mahogany wood and covered with gray chenille spreads like those in the Roosevelt Hotel where we were staying. A deaf-blind child walked aimlessly through the hallway, and partially sighted children led totally blind children to the dining room. Knowing that I could see, my parents anxiously wondered how this setting would affect me.

Mother was especially appalled to observe children eating on tin plates in the dining room. The staff explained that children moving silverware on tin plates could tell by sound if they were placing food on their forks.

After the director informed my parents that I could start any time, Mother vehemently refused to send me, explaining that she would see me only on weekends. The School for the Blind was approximately 300 miles from Alpena, Michigan.

"You don't have mother love, but smother love!" the director roared. "Apparently, her kindergarten teacher referred Sandra to MSB. If Sandy can't learn in a regular class, what alternative does she have?"

"I'll teach her myself!" Mother retorted. "You think I have smother love, but I believe that Sandy should attend school in her home environment where she belongs. Eventually, she will have to compete with normally sighted people. The sooner she does so, the better." When my parents met me after the tour to return home, I was angry and disappointed until Mother reassured me that things would work out after she talked with Mrs. Stone.

For six months, that director wrote to my parents, hounding them to enroll me at the Michigan School for the Blind, but they stuck to their guns, insisting that I attend Ella White School in Alpena.

Meanwhile, due to the power of prayer at St. Anne's Mother of Perpetual Help novenas and my parents' frequent conferences with Herbert Fox, the school principal, Mrs. Stone finally realized that I did not intend to disrupt the class while exploring my surroundings. We won round one of my many mainstreaming hurdles!

CHAPTER 4: CROSSING THE RUBICON INTO MAINSTREAMING

Following our hard-won victory with Mrs. Stone, more mainstreaming hurdles loomed ahead. Imagine living in a town of only 15,000 in the 1950s and 1960s as parents to the only visually impaired student attending a school system ill-equipped at the time to meet the needs of that student. Whom would they rely on for advice and inquire regarding obtaining special materials such as large-print textbooks? Without Dr. Ruedemann's guidance, Mother, indeed, would have been in a quandary. Serving as our valuable liaison, Dr. Ruedemann wrote letters to Ella White School, recommending that I be placed in a front seat near the blackboard and supplied with large-print textbooks which Mother had to purchase herself while I was in first through third grades.

Words cannot adequately express my gratitude toward my parents' active involvement in school activities, a significant building block to adjustment and well-being. If all parents demonstrated that commitment to their children's education, children would be more eager to learn and teachers more fulfilled. When Dad worked days, he and Mother always attended our evening school plays and concerts and chaperoned our seventh- and eighth-grade dances. They also helped Nancy and me with homework whenever necessary. Mother attended every parent-teacher conference, baked treats for school parties, purchased Christmas gifts for the elementary teachers, and arrived on visiting days.

I looked forward to visiting days at school, because I felt so proud of Mother when she entered the classroom. She was a classy lady, impeccably standing at 5 ft. petite, within pretty curviness. Her beautiful blue eyes readily appraised and changed color depending upon mood from deep indigo blue to almost violet. She usually wore multi-color floral pattern flared skirts with stiffly starched and crisply ironed white long-sleeved blouses or dresses with matching high-heeled shoes.

Visiting days gave each class an opportunity to showcase something outstanding, such as artwork, amazing somersaults in gym, even an eighth-grade mock court trial. For me, this usually meant a sample of improved handwriting on the bulletin board, a recently completed arithmetic assignment with an A on top, singing a song, or reciting poetry.

However, I must admit I misbehaved during a visiting day in kindergarten when Mrs. Stone was instructing her class to form a band playing with rhythm sticks, drums, triangles, and bells. Instead of shaking the bells I received, I shook my head and pouted, "I want a drum!" Apparently, Mrs. Stone had earmarked the drums for the boys.

Looking back, I can imagine Mother's violet eyes immediately shifting to storm clouds and her jaw dropping. Turning to me, she hissed, "Pay attention! Do as you're told, or you know what you'll get at home!" I shook the bells all right!

Though finally settling down to the class routine by first grade, initially I could not understand directions given by my teacher to the group unless they were given to me individually. Having difficulty printing within the lines, I had used yellow sight-saving paper with bold green lines, but do not remember how this paper was obtained.

Though the exception rather than the norm, teachers accommodated me in various ways. For example, knowing how copying addition and subtraction problems from the board would slow down my speed during tests, Mrs. Schiller, my second-grade teacher, gave me mimeographed copies of these problems. Also noticing my difficulty distinguishing one inch from half and quarter inches on a ruler, she drew a larger ruler on the blackboard for me to use until I was able to transfer the skill in reading that ruler to the regular print ones used in class.

During third grade, successful mainstreaming also meant effectively asserting myself against the playground hellions who often instigated snowball fights and broke Nancy's glasses. Knowing that I did not see well, they often teased me. "Want some peanuts, Sandy?" Upon opening their offering, out popped a real looking snake! They also made paper wads and snapped them on my ears, sneaked behind me, roaring like lions, barking like vicious dogs, and tripping me while catching me off guard.

Mrs. Gapczynski taught me an indelible lesson in tough love. Instead of excusing me from recess, she confronted me, "How will you handle it?"

"Nancy will protect me."

"Oh, come on, Sandy! Nancy would want to play with her own chums at recess. Remember, when you go through life, you'll have to fight your own battles, because she won't always be around to protect you."

Armed with Dad's pep talk, "Don't take any guff," acute hearing, and uncanny sound localization in my arsenal, I reached up, grabbed, and tore the paper wads every time they snapped alongside my ears. Whenever the offenders attempted to trip me, I surprised them with a combination-style bear hug and python squeeze. I also mimicked their animal noises. Soon the boys tired of their game and left me alone.

That year, I also reached a milestone in reading regular print. Curiously leafing through a classmate's copy of *The New Friends and Neighbors* reader, I noticed that his book included colored pictures depicting real-life representations of people, buildings, plants, and animals instead of mine which only contained blank drawings on pastel colored paper. To my amazement, I could read the smaller print by holding the book up close to my eyes. When I read out of that book, Mrs. Gapczynski marveled, "I never knew you could read small print! How wonderful!" From then on, I received regular print readers like the other children.

Miss Doris Eva, my fourth-grade teacher who complimented me on "singing exceptionally well" on my report cards and Miss Lightbody, the music teacher, both nurtured my inherent love for music. Coordinating all plays held at Ella White School during American Education Week in November, Miss Lightbody selected me for character roles or solos, all of which I relished except the beginning of one hair-raising solo within a fourth-grade western play. An electrical shock surged through me as I held the microphone. If I continued to hold the microphone, I would fry, and if I dropped it, it would thunder on the floor. Noticing my dilemma, the stage-hand immediately closed the curtain and offered me another microphone. Not missing a beat, I continued singing and received thunderous applause.

In fifth grade, much to Mrs. Stahl's consternation, my interest in her Bible lessons, deemed vital as the three R's and conducted from the time she taught in a rural school, paled in comparison with my passion for music. Since I did not understand Scriptures, my boredom with them led me to a more entertaining diversion of disassembling my ball point pens, setting up their parts like imaginary bowling pins on my desktop, and knocking them over with the pen filters.

After Mrs. Stahl informed Mother of this misbehavior during parent-teacher conference, Mother advised me, "Show the same respect toward her daily Bible readings as you do when you pledge allegiance to the flag, even though the psalms may be difficult to understand."

Finishing a reading in *Our Daily Bread* about a first-grade teacher who made the class recite the 23rd Psalm, I realized how Mrs. Stahl had tried to scatter the seeds of God's love as that first-grade teacher had done. Perhaps on earth and in heaven, she has persistently prayed for a mischievous sinner like me to be drawn into the fold. Little did she dream how these seeds would eventually blossom into my yearning for the Word as an adult.

Simply expecting me to complete the tests within the time limits allowed, teachers advised me to concentrate on getting as many correctly done as possible. Praying, "Jesus mercy, Mary help," before tests relaxed me and increased my concentration. Dogged fear of appearing stupid in class if I consistently scored low, as well as personal pride when I scored high, impelled me to study hard and to do my best on tests.

I excelled in English, French, and arithmetic but floundered in geography, history, geometry, and science classes. Though flourishing in spelling, essay and report writing, memorization, reading comprehension, and class discussion, I withered while drawing and interpreting maps, graphs, tables, timelines, plant and animal cells, science experiments, and bisecting angles. I could not have managed without Nancy's and Dad's help in completing these assignments.

Reflecting on teachers' attitudes toward mainstreaming and learning, I salute Mr. Roderick Magoon, my eighth-grade science teacher and the impetus behind this book! As my hero, he embodied dedication and passion for his subject and students, creativity, and daring while attempting innovative teaching methods in the face of skepticism. Being perceptive, he realized challenges I would face as the only visually impaired student in class.

Unlike other science teachers who compelled us to replicate drawings of plant or animal cells presented in our textbooks or memorize and regurgitate irrelevant material on tests, Roderick involved the whole class through interactive participation in WFF'N PROOF games to develop skills in thinking logically and in problem solving. His motto was, "Be alert, not inert!" Completing stimulating projects and giving presentations, we experienced a hands-on practical and engaging learning approach to science. Examples of class projects I completed included a report on milkweed; a well-balanced dinner menu plan categorizing food into fats, proteins, carbohydrates, and starches; and breaking them down into vitamins and calories. For the electricity unit, Dad helped me design an apparatus displaying a circuit tester with an accompanying description of its function.

Roderick assigned each student the granddaddy of challenges over Christmas vacation to research and write a report about 100 machines, their operation, and contribution to civilization. Shortly after the whole class handed in this homework, Roderick Magoon summoned Nancy and me to see him after class. "Didn't I assign you a report on 100 machines?" he sternly reprimanded us. "I suspect that you were cheating because I noticed conspicuous duplication on both of your papers. I have no choice but to give you both a failing grade." After we arrived home late for lunch and tearfully explained to her what had happened, Mother descended upon Ella White

School and Mr. Magoon, "You mean to tell me that with twin daughters living in the same house, you would not expect a certain degree of duplication?" Fortunately for Nancy and me, Roderick reversed his decision to flunk us and never again referred to that incident during the remainder of that year.

In addition to projects, Roderick assigned each student a five-minute presentation on science topics every grading period. At the beginning of my first speech, I became extremely nervous and apologized for it. Taking me aside afterwards, Roderick advised me to know my material and never to apologize while giving presentations. Eventually, I improved with his encouragement. This exemplifies how Roderick motivated all his students to do their best by maximizing their strengths and the philosophy, "Practice makes perfect" to minimize their weaknesses.

As life ebbs and flows like the tides, Nancy and I never fathomed that Roderick Magoon's and our paths would once again cross 47 years later via his internet address, eventually leading to regular emails. After teaching science in 1962 and 44 years of English and creative writing, Roderick has pursued writing as a self-satisfying hobby, having prolifically written short stories, and a handful of novels including *Life with Larry*. In fact, during the summer of 2009, Roderick suggested, "You have a way with words. Why don't you share your experiences and insights about blindness into a book?"

He discussed subjects with depth, warmth, and witty satire. For this and other reasons mentioned in this chapter, knowing him has inspired and enriched my life. I certainly miss him as a teacher and a friend since his passing in 2017.

CHAPTER 5: AN IOTA OF IDYLLIC ICONS

After cable television was finally installed on our block during the autumn of 1958, Nancy and I sat riveted to suspenseful *Bonanza*, *Gun Smoke*, and *Rawhide* episodes of sheriffs nabbing outlaws and marveled at Perry Mason's and Joe Friday's facility in winning trials and cracking cases. I also recall, while growing up, a dearth of stories about blind people represented in literature, on TV, and in movies. For example, the only story about a blind person that I remember in the lower grades was about a boy accidentally blinded when he carelessly played with firecrackers. Had I read Laura Ingalls Wilder's entire Little House series or watched too many TV episodes of *Little House on the Prairie*, I would have found Mary's resignation to sitting in a rocking chair all day as depressing as Selina D'Arcy's confinement in her grandfather's tenement apartment in *A Patch of Blue*. Rejecting that kind of lifestyle, I strove to emulate the strong and able-bodied, because, as I reasoned, they had more control over their lives. Since people esteemed them, I assumed only they could be heroes. Otherwise, who would admire a weakling?

Living in Alpena, I only knew of a handful of blind people, including Peter Gillard, a boy my age who attended the Michigan School for the Blind; Sally Lappan, a curator at Holy Cross Cemetery in Alpena; and Agnes McGillivery, an elderly neighbor, blind due to diabetes, who fondly reminisced about making samplers when she could see. Mother also mentioned that a Mr. Bill McGurn, a blind man who earned his living by singing at weddings and funerals, beautifully sang Franz Schubert's

"Ave Maria" at Uncle Joe's funeral. Though three other partially sighted students attended Alpena Community College with me, I did not chum closely with them since they took different courses and stayed in the dorm while I lived at home.

At first, I did not regard any of these people as significant role models, except Grandma Foster (surname Anglicized from "Fortier" to "Foster" for easier pronunciation), Dad's French-Canadian mother who became blind later in life due to diabetes. Grandma looked like a typical 1950s diminutive 5' 2" grandmother with same-style straight, below-the- knee, long-sleeve dresses, either navy blue or black, with big buttons down the front or huge bows under the collar in contrast to the severity of the style. She wore orthopedic lace-up black shoes with a small heel. She was bespectacled with grey hair fashioned in a bun at the back of her neck. She was very plain in features but beautiful in warmth and heart.

Grandma Foster, a quiet, soft-spoken lady, never complained. She often babysat with Nancy and me while Mother and Dad grocery shopped at Midway Supermarket and always invited us to join her for dinner afterwards which usually consisted of crepes served with salmon and vinegar sauce since we as Catholics had to abstain from eating meat on Fridays.

She should have been canonized as a saint after taking care of me while Nancy in 1952 underwent surgery for strabismus, or crossed eyes, at Harper Hospital in Detroit. I do not know how Grandma tolerated my incessant, "When are Mom and Nancy coming home?" "In a few minutes," she replied patiently. Lonesome and unable to understand the procedure of surgery and recovery, I threw tantrums, because Mother did not return home immediately.

Being deeply religious, Grandma Foster fervently prayed and tried to teach Nancy and me the Hail Mary and Our Father in French, but we were too young to understand the language. Realizing this, Grandma encouraged us to pray with her in English.

Grandma Foster always enjoyed accompanying our family on picnics and Sunday drives and treating us to ice cream cones or "combs" as she pronounced the "m." Though she and I spent most of the time sleeping in the back seat during the drive-in movie, togetherness mattered most to her regardless of the activity. Though Grandma has been gone for many years now, I still miss her and admire her for her steadfast faith in Jesus and the Blessed Virgin Mary. What beautiful memories she has left behind for me to cherish!

When I was in fifth grade, Mother read an article in the *Grit Magazine* about Anne Wiegand, a visually impaired senior at Short Ridge High School in Indianapolis, Indiana, who aspired to teach blind children. Since I, too, was interested in that career, Mother encouraged me to write to Anne which continued for about a year until she stopped writing to me. Whether she fulfilled her dream I will never know.

Reading history textbooks extolling the wealthy and the famous but not representing blind people distressed me during the 1950s and 1960s. Didn't God endow both blind and sighted with special attributes and talents?

However, an emotional turning point arose for me during a field trip to the Alpena Public Library when our sixth-grade teacher assigned the class to write reports on historical contributions to society. Voilà! How excited I was when I discovered a book about Louis Braille, a French child whose accidental blindness compelled him to invent an alphabet enabling the blind to read and write!

He eventually taught at the Royal Institute for the Blind in Paris where he attended as a child. His students admired him as a teacher and a friend. In fact, he mentored former classmates when they became apprentice teachers at the Institute. He even purchased books, slates, and styluses, and established scholarships for needy students. Enchanted with his life, I decided to write a composition about him.

Louis Braille's compassion and alphabet, which had generated those educational and employment opportunities for blind children in nineteenth century France, stimulated me to question, "How can I nobly contribute to society?" After I expressed this aspiration to Mother, she pondered for a while and then stated, "Any good deed pleases God. It doesn't matter if it's great or small. Though it may not be as famous as Louis Braille's alphabet, you can continue helping the needy significantly with your donations to the Salvation Army Christmas kettle. You started that when you were five years old. I'm proud of your concern for others, and I encourage that."

Yet something gnawed at me. Admiring how unselfishly Louis Braille reached out to poor blind students motivated me to give more generously to the needy than only donating to the Salvation Army kettles. That opportunity arrived sooner than I had expected.

After noticing an ad in *The Alpena News* an hour later, Mother suggested another idea. "Hey, girls! Let's enter the Midway Supermarket raffle! If we win the turkey, we can give it to a poor family at Christmas." To our surprise, we won!

One of my classmates came from a poor family of eight children who lived on an isolated rural road ten miles from Alpena. She always wore hand-me-downs and gym shoes instead of boots in the winter.

On Christmas Eve day, Mother, our neighbor Catherine and her children, Nancy, and I packed boxes of outgrown toys and clothes, and enough non-perishable food for a lavish Christmas feast and leftovers thereafter. Then we all piled into Catherine's station wagon headed toward that classmate's home. Soon we stopped at a yellow wooden framed house with peeling paint, several shingles blown off the roof, and porch steps full of gaping holes akin to a mouthful of missing teeth.

How shocked we were when we entered! Even their windows covered with plastic layers could not prevent drafts. The family owned a pot belly stove in the living room as the only source of heat. An afghan covered a moth-eaten mohair couch. Threadbare throw rugs lay on the wooden floor. The whole place smelled of mustiness and fried potatoes.

As soon as we placed the boxes on the table, the children gleefully tugged at the packages. Their parents shook their heads in disbelief then hugged us tightly. I do not know who reacted more joyfully, the family or us. Reading an inspirational story acted as a catalyst in creating a cherished childhood Christmas memory which evolved into our family tradition of donating Thanksgiving baskets and Christmas gifts for the needy.

Seeing *The Miracle Worker* in 1962 and reading Helen Keller's *The Story of My Life* a year later for an English class also filled me with elation and admiration. Helen Keller fascinated me, since her autobiography showcases a warm, vibrant person centered in a vivid tapestry of memories appealing to all senses. In photographs, she also impressed me as a poised woman, a quality that is still a work in progress for me.

Considering Helen Keller's struggles replaced self-pity with intense appreciation for my senses of hearing and even partial sight. Until then I felt deprived. Comparing myself to Nancy in childhood reinforced this feeling. Shame on me!

At least I could speak, for example, but Helen had to communicate using sign language. Whereas Helen learned to identify objects through touch and colors by mentally associating them with objects, I could see colors and objects up close to identify them. While a student at Cambridge School for Young Ladies and Radcliff College, Helen could only obtain lecture and textbook materials through Anne Sullivan's spelling the words verbatim into her hand. On the other hand, I could reread lessons to understand concepts, hear teachers' instructions and lectures, take notes, and participate directly in class discussions. Thereafter, I chose Helen Keller as a model in resilience.

Noting Anne Sullivan's extraordinary patience, dedication, flexibility, and confidence in Helen's ability to learn, I would strive to emulate these qualities as a successful future teacher. In fact, I often fantasized being a contemporary Anne Sullivan as an adult.

As a youth, I could identify with Anne Sullivan's blindness and resolution, but in some respects, I had difficulty relating to her because of our age differences and the sharp contrasts in our lifestyles. Yet her childhood intrigued me because of its contrasts to mine. Reading about Anne Sullivan's life in the Tewksbury Almshouse aroused my curiosity about the interior of asylums during the 1800s and empathy regarding treatment of inmates. Again, this reminded me how much I had taken my blessings for granted.

As much as I revered Grandma Foster, Louis Braille, Helen Keller, and Anne Sullivan, a new icon soon captured my interest and heart—Stevie Wonder! One could have labeled me as a star-struck fourteen-year-old in

1963 when his "Fingertips" topped the charts. At last, a teen-age idol with whom I could identify as a blind person! Imagine his overcoming blindness, poverty, and racism! His unique, catchy music fascinated me and sent me gyrating. I faithfully listened to his records played every night on Record Roundup more than the other pop stars' records the previous year and watched him on the Ed Sullivan Show.

Mother and Dad even reacted with a mixture of amusement and surprise. "What gives? We thought you enjoyed classical music!"

"Mom, when you were my age, you had Glenn Miller, Guy Lombardo, and Les Brown," I retorted.

Louis Braille, Helen Keller, Anne Sullivan, and Stevie Wonder showed me how other blind people adapted to relying on their remaining senses. Nor was I the only blind person ridiculed or crammed into a narrow niche. Like these heroes, I would not allow blindness to define my life, either.

Knowing a creative, just, and a loving God, I believe that He would be immensely proud of Grandma Foster, Louis Braille, Anne Sullivan, Helen Keller, and Stevie Wonder. This includes Helen Keller's mentor Alexander Graham Bell and Stevie Wonder's tutor Ted Hull. They all served humanity without seeking renown, as God had instructed His apostles in Mark 10:43 and Matthew 20:26. These icons' zeal to make the world a better place melded into God's vision of service exemplifying greatness.

Illustrating the parable of the mustard seed according to Mathew 13:31-32, stories of my chosen role models revealed their suspected nil or untapped potential for success which ultimately flourished through His grace into huge plants bearing the fruit of their marvelous accomplishments. Rainbows of hope emanating from these stories dissipated my countless feelings of ineptitude.

Reflecting on these scriptures of Mark and Matthew presented during a homily when I was young, I also began noting Sally Lappan's and Mr. McGurn's inherently positive influence upon other Alpena residents. God blessed them, too, with their own special abilities. Curator of Holy Cross Cemetery did not initially correspond with my sixth-grade conception of a spectacular role.

As time went on, I recognized that Sally's years of employment there spoke volumes. Her pleasant personality attracted many people. She rented her own apartment and always rode her bike to and from work. Though I did not know Mr. McGurn personally, I could say that he glorified God by singing for numerous weddings and funerals. How I wish I had heard him singing Schubert's "Ave Maria" in a spellbinding performance!

Analyzing the lives of blind people chosen as my role models while growing up taught me that greatness embodies altruism, moral character, imagination, motivation, mentorship, integrity, and responsibility in thought and action. I also learned that potential for greatness is both inherent and acquired and that greatness, unlike fame, is immortal.

CHAPTER 6: AT THE THRESHOLD

What a year of milestones! Our parents celebrated our thirteenth birthday by converting unnecessary storage space upstairs into a bedroom, half bath, and study for my sister and me. They painted our walls white and purchased white bedspreads with red and pink hearts. Finally, a quiet retreat in which to pray, study, read, and even daydream! I hated studying on the kitchen table because of the frequent interruptions when visitors arrived. Mom and Dad, too, often forfeited TV viewing until our homework was done.

As another milestone, Nancy and I began wearing nylons and fancy flats to church and other dressy occasions. Mother asserted we would graduate to high heels later even though we clamored for them then.

We idolized the latest pop singers and eagerly listened to their Top Ten Hits on Record Roundup when we finished our homework. Our favorites were "Soldier Boy," "Johnny Get Angry," "Speedy Gonzales," and "Now Do the Twist."

Now that Nancy and I were growing up and eager to expand our horizons, our family summer vacations combined more history and culture with fun. While vacationing in Mackinac Island, we often rode the carriages, gaped at the Grand Hotel, and frequented many fudge and souvenir shops! When my parents weren't looking, I peeked into other smaller hotels lining the sidewalks. What stories would they tell? One hotel bragged of a staircase with a curving banister and French doors.

Student performances of symphony and choral concerts mesmerized me for hours during a family tour of

Interlochen Arts Academy. How I wished I then had souvenir recordings of choirs and orchestras!

Nancy and I especially recall the teenaged excitement of the July, 1962, trip to Boblo Island, Canada with Aunt Helen and Uncle Harold and our wait in line with the three young guys who reminded us of the actors who played in Evan Hunter's book *A Matter of Conviction* and the movie, "The Young Savages." *A Matter of Conviction* was the first book we ever bought off a rack at Sepull's drugstore after we saw the movie. Mom had Dad preview it before she would let us read it.

We can still remember the balmy warm night, pleasant smells of summer, the Big Band music wafting through the air and lazily relaxing on the ferry deck, watching the middle-age/elderly couples dancing cheek-to-cheek on the wooden dance floor. Dad, Uncle Harry, and I rode the Mighty Mouse, one of the daring-do roller coaster rides. Mother joked, "Watching the three of you on the ride was worth buying the ticket." I think Uncle Harry who was in his late fifties then may have outdone himself!

That weekend, our visit to Greenfield Village in Dearborn, Michigan showcased its antique cars, farm implements, and furniture. Until then, history had never appealed to me, as it merely consisted of memorizing dates and drawing maps. However, Abraham Lincoln's chair in Ford Theater the night he was assassinated, replicas of slave cabins and pioneer villages transformed history from a dull subject into an interesting one.

Writing articles for the monthly school newspaper *The Flash* highlighted my eighth-grade year. I wrote an article about a principal's tour of Cobo Hall in Detroit, Michigan. Shortly after, I interviewed and wrote other articles featuring students who achieved special awards. Working on the class prophecy, we devised some humorous predictions. Imagine me being a co-owner of a bowling alley with another classmate!

As another cherry on the sundae, Miss Howard, our gym teacher, offered me a trophy for improved average attained while bowling on the after-school Friday Girls' Athletic Association league. The trophy made from a bowling pin had a face consisting of a wig styled in a ponytail and little glasses. My average started at 69 and improved to 135.

The day of our eighth-grade graduation dance, Nancy and I got our hair done in a ratted, bouffant style. That evening we felt grown up in our pastel blue dresses over billowing slips and matching shoes. Time sped by while we danced as did that year.

At summer's end, I eagerly and nervously anticipated high school. Unlike Ella White Elementary, which was constructed on one floor, Alpena High, an older cream stucco building, consisted of three stories. Therefore, as I was informed during freshman orientation and registration, attending classes required climbing three flights of stairs with only five minutes between classes.

The locker combination presented a problem during orientation. Not knowing how to operate one and having considerable difficulty reading the small numbers on the lock, how would I handle this?

Through practice, I learned to open a larger combination lock at home. Meeting two days later with the principal, Mother and I requested substituting that large-print combination lock, but that proved impossible. Even if the original combination lock were removed, no other sized combination lock could fit in the hole. Lugging all books to classes would have been the only other alternative. How about this for developing muscles?

I should not have worried. The first day, I easily opened my locker and punctually arrived for classes, except for algebra. After I apologized for being late, Mr. Foster smiled, "That's to be expected."

I had the front seat near the blackboard, but other accommodations remained the exception at Alpena High as they did in grade school. One history teacher read items for me from transparencies displayed on the overhead projector and filmstrip captions. The biology teacher excused me from drawing pictures of cells. "Just study the diagrams in your book," he instructed. After I singed my bangs while putting my face too close to observe a candle the first day in chemistry class, Mr. Adolf Brosz kept me under his radar and assigned me a lab assistant during every experiment. Miraculously, the chemistry lab did not explode!

The Mixed Chorus and the Girls' Choir directors insisted that everybody sight read the music. I circumvented this dilemma by pretending to read the music while I memorized the notes played on the piano.

As in elementary school, teachers expected me to complete exams and homework within the stipulated time
frames.

Wanting to be like other students, I enrolled in physical education and swimming, though I must admit being
klutzy in gym. One day, for example, while attempting a
basic balancing pose on the pommel horse, I resembled
the listing *Titanic*. Forget about progressing to circles
on the horse as the class objective! Instead of slowly dis-
mounting as Mrs. Van Natter had instructed, I rambunc-
tiously jumped from the horse and fell, breaking my big
right toe. Thank heavens Dad was working a shift that
allowed him to drive me back and forth to school that
week!

During the next several months, I also created some
modern dance movements to a lively piece, "The Bull-
fight." My Paso Dobles would not have garnered the
"weapon of mass seduction" award from Dancing with
the Stars judges nor would my playing the matador have
incited a bull to charge. In retrospect, if I were given
the choice of swimming over physical education during
freshman year, I would have preferred swimming.

Apparently, the long-ago effort of passing advanced
beginner swimming with Mr. Gillespie paid off. He and
Miss Leonall, my freshman swimming instructor, invited
me to participate in a demonstration on teaching swimming to special needs children held at Alpena High
School pool. How proud I was initially!

This demonstration consisted of an out-of-town instructor and three other teenagers, one developmentally disabled and two with cerebral palsy. Uncle Evans, as
he liked to be called, asked each of us to pretend that
she was a particular dog and to show him how she would
swim. Believing that Uncle Evans should have inquired
about more age-appropriate interests, such as school,
swimming goals, or hobbies, I inwardly chafed at this
juvenile activity. If other adults expected us to behave
maturely regardless of our disabilities, why didn't he?
Perhaps, he assumed that since we could not function
well physically, we could not think or carry on intelligent
conversations. Were those other teenagers functioning
at a lower cognitive level than I realized? Did he relate
better to children than to teenagers or adults?

On the drive home, Mother asked me, "Why did you initially recoil from Uncle Evans when he told you to feel his motions during the back stroke? You performed the other strokes beautifully after he showed you how to do them."

"Mom, I didn't want to go near him, because his breath reeked of alcohol."

"What! Had we known that we wouldn't let you participate."

Fortunately, my participation offered Miss Leonall valuable insight in teaching with hands-on instruction. This, in turn, offered me the opportunity to meet other special needs students and to improve my swimming techniques and stamina.

Contrasting with Ella White School, the high-school world expanded with students transferred from surrounding Sanborn Township, Alpena public schools including Ella White, Bingham, Lincoln, Hinks, and McPhee. Here I felt like a fish swiftly swept from a small pond into ocean waves. Unaware of my visual problems I shamefully concealed, students had regarded me as standoffish when I passed them in the halls without greeting them. Had I explained my situation to them, perhaps they would have reacted empathetically, but I'm looking through a rearview mirror. Feeling awkward about talking to people and introducing myself, I mostly stood as a wallflower at school dances. How happy I was when someone did ask me to dance!

Requiring more time to complete homework than it did other students seldom left me with enough time for extracurricular activities. Deeply concerned, the high-school principal congratulated me for being on the semester honor roll but added that participating in extracurricular activities as well as academic achievement developed more well-rounded students. Heeding his advice, I did participate in Mixed Chorus, the French and the Future Teachers' Clubs, and Girls' Choir. Since football huddles scrambled into blurry bodies and the excitement of merely hearing the crowd cheer our team's touchdowns wore off after a while, I preferred basketball games to football games. Sitting close to even one basket gave me a splendid close-up view of the action.

During the spring of 1964, a guidance counselor coordinated a summer driver's education class for high-school students 15 years of age and over. Aware of my visual limitations, she pooh-poohed my enrollment in driver's education. When I returned home from school blubbering, Mother scolded, "You sign up even if I have to go with you! Don't be afraid of her. Speak up! Tell her how you never begged off gym because of poor eyesight. Why not drive?" Mother knew her psychology of playing upon the typical teenage embarrassment of being seen with parents by peers. This motivated me to assert myself. During one week of class, I scored 80-90% on quizzes over chapters read nightly but did not pass the eye or the simulated driving tests.

"Aw shucks!" I thought," While other teenagers will have their licenses, I'll still be riding my bike!" The school nurse's comment, "You must realize there are certain things you will be unable to do in life," did not mitigate the disappointment of failing this teenage rite of passage. To console me, Dad gave me the feel of driving on isolated country roads. In fact, I quickly caught on to the stick shift on the steering column, loved to speed and hear gravel fly over the tires. Experiencing the white-knuckled ride of her life, Mother shrieked, "Sandy!" Dad laughed, "Am I glad Sandy isn't driving because my insurance rates would fly through the roof!"

That summer, Dr. Ruedemann encouraged me to consider college seriously. Believing that I would qualify for one, he began investigating available college scholarships after the eye appointment was over.

At the Alpena Armory staged Battles of the Bands, Nancy and I always looked forward to voting for the best band. I enjoyed them more than dances at school. Though teenagers danced to records during bands' breaks, the performances occupying most of the evenings spared me the wallflower awkwardness of freshman year.

Nancy and I remember the first time we walked from home and ventured up the steps into unknown maturity. At first, we escaped into the ladies' room to catch our breath for a while but hearing the great music and feeling the beat finally gave us courage to venture onto the dance floor with those older strangers.

Mother correctly assumed that I really went to the Armory to see the groups' funny get-ups rather than hear the music. Somehow, I maneuvered to stand close enough to the stage to see them. For instance, the Sir Douglas Quintet wore rather heavy furry, nondescript-colored tunics. That group with shoulder length hair appeared as a cross between the Rolling Stones and the Kinks. While performing, including their signature song, "Are You a Boy?" the Barbarians dressed like pirates with eye patches, blue jeans, sandals, and leather vests over cream shirts. Moulty, the lead singer who wore a hook, performed a tear-jerking song he composed about how he lost his left hand playing with a homemade bomb as a boy. His last words especially tugged at my heart, "If I had a girl, my life would be complete." The Count and the Colony wore plaid suits with white ruffled shirts and hats like those worn by Paul Revere. I admired the shimmering gowns of the Crystals.

To offset the disappointment of not driving, adolescent loneliness, and low self-esteem, I participated with the Girls' Choir in a Michigan Choral Festival at Catholic Central High School. On that March 27, 1965 Saturday morning after we attended adjudication of singing three choral pieces, "Oh, Love Deep as the River," "Snow Legend," and "Clouds," and sight reading, we received a rating of "one" on our songs but a rating of "five" (poor) on sight reading.

After lunch, the Alpena High School Girls' Choir and mixed a cappella choir joined the other participating Michigan high school choirs in a mass concert of two numbers, a patriotic piece and "The Banana Boat Song." I was exhilarated to sing at the Michigan Choral Festival, in school assemblies, Christmas, and spring concerts, and at graduation Class Nights.

As another self-esteem booster, summer employment in 1965 initially consisted of feeding the neighbor's rabbits while he and his family were on vacation. Nancy and I had enough of babysitting after one day. Volunteering at Pied Piper Center for developmentally disabled children and adults consisted of working with them once a week on social interaction, playing table games for recreation, and helping with the Pied Piper benefit car wash. Although I think we got more suds on us than on the cars we washed, we did have fun.

During one eventful border crossing upon returning from the Canadian Soo into Michigan during the summer of 1966, my family and I successfully smuggled

39

forbidden fireworks that we had purchased by hiding them in our luggage. Going through customs, of course, required maintaining strict poker faces. This was challenging since I am a poor liar, but I pulled it off. The neighbors must have jealously marveled at our fireworks extravaganza that Fourth of July. Otherwise, the summer went by uneventfully, because I could not find summer employment that suited my abilities.

During that summer, Nancy and I learned a lesson about deferred versus immediate gratification. Having spent all our money on lesser-known bands, we were keenly disappointed when we discovered that Sonny and Cher were going to be in Alpena and Mother was unwilling to subsidize us. Though we did not see Sonny and Cher, we had attended and enjoyed other concerts at the Armory with other named bands, such as the Guess Who, a Canadian folk/rock group.

Dr. Ruedemann was concerned when I informed him during my July, 1966, visit about the heavy volume of reading required for my upcoming senior English, history, and civics courses. To ensure their prompt arrival, he immediately ordered textbooks for me in talking book media from the Library of Congress and the Michigan Library for the Blind and Physically Handicapped. He also informed me that he would continue laying the groundwork for my college scholarship through the Department of Services for the Blind in Alpena.

Later that fall, Nancy and I took our SAT exams. Instead of requiring that I take the Saturday SAT with the group, my high school counselor administered the large-print SAT at home on Thursday, November 3, 1966, as an accommodation. Since classes were canceled anyway due to the winter weather advisory, I could not understand why he gave me the test from 6 p.m. until midnight instead of earlier in the day when I was more mentally refreshed. His over-the-shoulder presence from the beginning of the exam to the end making sure I did not cheat racked both my nerves and concentration. A month later, I was notified of my poor performance, 80% on the verbal and 60% in the mathematics/science portion of the SAT.

The following January, Nancy and I applied to Alpena Community College and took the required college physical exam. Since Alpena had no community mental health agency, I was also scheduled to complete a psychological evaluation in February at the State Hospital in Traverse City, Michigan. To qualify for the Services for the Blind scholarship, I had to complete this assessment determining if I had an adequate IQ for college level work. The drive there filled me with intense apprehension of wondering what careers I would pursue if I did not pass.

When one friendly psychologist questioned me regarding my feelings about young adulthood and career aspirations, I replied that I was looking forward to attending college, because I wanted to teach visually impaired children. When he asked me if I dated, I quipped, "No. But oh, if I could see well, I'd be a better flirt!" He later informed my parents, "Other than her limited vision, she is normal!"

Dr. Bierce, a metallic-voiced psychologist, administered the Wechsler Adult Intelligence Scale (WAIS) orally as the reasonable accommodation then for the blind. I was later informed that I attained an IQ score of 122 in the superior range.

On March 13, 1967, the move from the old high school on Second Avenue occurred to the new high school on 3303 South Third, uprooting everyone, especially seniors longing to have graduated from the old high school. Riding to school because of heavy traffic and no sidewalks, Nancy and I missed walking with our friends. All students were only allowed to eat lunch in their respective commons. Nancy's and my only enjoyment of the day was eating Mother's most delicious meatloaf, roast beef, or chicken sandwiches.

Finally, the long-awaited graduation week arrived in a whirl of celebrations. On June 5, 1967, the Alpena Rotary Club hosted a noon luncheon at the Civic Center honoring all Alpena High and Catholic Central High School seniors who achieved cum laude status. Later that evening, Alpena High School graduates attended a buffet dinner at Lake Winyah Club, accompanied by a band playing elegant dinner music including "Summertime" and "Some Enchanted Evening."

I dreaded attending the upcoming June 6 Class of '67 Senior Awards Night. Brooding over my lack of popularity in high school and disappointment of barely missing the National Honor Society. I dawdled until Mother burst into my room. "What's the matter with you tonight?"

"I just don't have the heart to participate in tonight's activities. Nobody likes me. Nobody will even miss me, so why bother?"

"Sandy, someday you'll regret it if you don't participate in the ceremonies tonight. Now hurry up and finish getting dressed."

Later as the list of students receiving class night awards droned on and on, I wanted all this to end, wishing that I were in my bedroom. Much to my astonishment, I heard my name called. In what seemed like a dream, I slowly made my way to the podium where Mr. Finch, the school principal, presented me with my scholarship through the Department of Services for the Blind.

As I returned to my seat, I was further astonished to hear applause that shook the room. Suddenly, I felt and heard the audience stand up as one. They were giving me a standing ovation! Little did I dream I would receive anything like that!

The motivational commencement speech of June 8 electrified me. "Do you have the TIGER in you? You must have the TIGER in you to succeed!

T—Tenacity

I—Instinct in choosing the right vocational path and goals and in making the right decisions

G—Grit

E—Energy

R—Robustness in health and in tackling any challenge."

This message applies today as it did in 1967.

The exhilaration climaxed with the march on stage to receive our diplomas, accompanied by thunderous applause from the audience and the high school band playing "To Dream the Impossible Dream" from *Man of LaMancha.*

Besser Manufacturing Company's strike from the end of April to the beginning of October leaving Dad out of work impelled me to seek summer employment. On Friday following high school graduation, I inquired about possible jobs at Alpena Community College. Since they had available openings for cleaning aids during the summer, I requested an interview scheduled on the following Monday, June 12. During the interview, I mentioned that though I was short on experience, I was long on conscientiousness and work ethic. To my surprise, I was informed to report to work the next day.

During the summer of 1967, we also had fun with a little black 1960 Renault Dauphine with rusty, cream wheels and hubcaps that Nancy bought for $300 with the money she earned at Cooperative Extension Agency. Mother suggested painting the wheels yellow with left-over Sherwin Williams house paint. How we loved driving around listening to the radio blaring popular songs such as the Music Explosions' "A Little Bit o' Soul," The Doors' "Light my Fire," and The Troggs' "Wild Thing"! Some of the boys jokingly called our Renault "the pregnant roller skate."

Being more empathetic of my limited vision than high school students, Alpena Community College students helped me by giving me constructive criticism on speeches and taking lecture notes. More fellows asked me to dance. I also enjoyed attending the Alpena Civic Theater plays.

I thrived on class discussion but took notes in longhand. The bulky reel-to-reel tape recorder which the Department of Services for the Blind purchased challenged my strength as I lugged it from class to class. I hardly used it.

I also requested the front seat near the blackboard and that instructors read material from overhead projectors for me to take notes. In fact, after finishing their lectures, several instructors gave me their overheads. As in elementary and high school, instructors expected me to complete timed tests and homework promptly.

As a more technically savvy college student given expansive choices of technology and low vision devices available today, I would request financial aid for a computer and magnification computer software, such as Magic and ZoomText, which I had used at work as well as investigating reproduction of texts on e-Books and in digital recordings. Furthermore, I would also specify audio and large-print materials, as well as reasons for their need in writing before the beginning of each new semester. On the contrary in 1968, I was grateful to receive my own Smith Corona manual typewriter for college equipment.

When we met Barb Nisky and Sue Klien at Alpena Community College, how we enjoyed pizza at Odie's on Chisholm Street after Alpena Community College dances and going on explorations with Barb who always had "wheels!"

On August 17, 1968, at the Alpena County Fair, we ran into Ohio National Guards, one of which Barb knew from summer tour before. Then we went bowling. Experiencing a fluke, I scored 145!

On September 1, 1968, a horrible rainy day, we went to Mackinac Island where we spent more time drying out in souvenir shops and toured Mackinac College.

From April 7-9, 1969, Barb, Sue, Nancy, and I took a trip to Michigan State University to scout the campus and housing. Nancy and I liked the ivy-league old look of Yakeley, but Barb and Sue opted for the newer dorms on campus. The weather was so beautiful with spring flowers and flowering trees and warmer temperatures downstate and people in shirtsleeves rather than sweaters.

Amid the high jinks of sophomore year lay more serious issues of applying to Michigan State and for housing, graduation from Alpena Community College, again taking college physical exams, finding summer employment, and orientation to MSU. To my dismay, the library aide position I had held during July 1-August 31, 1968, at Alpena Community College was already filled. Lynn Hanisko, my Department of Services for the Blind rehabilitation counselor from fall 1968 to spring 1969, telephoned me on June 2, 1969, suggesting that I work during the summer as an aide at Pied Piper Center, beginning on June 16 and ending July 31, 1969, Mondays through Thursdays.

How I balked at first, wanting to teach blind children, not developmentally disabled ones! Within ten minutes, Lynn sped into our driveway, sprinted up our front steps, and then plunked himself at our kitchen table where he discussed this summer employment program with my parents and me. Thankfully, he did not tell me to go to Holy Hannah or else my stubbornness would have cost me this opportunity. While working with developmentally disabled children and adults, I could take a course, "The Exceptional Child," concurrently offered at Pied Piper Center as a satellite of Central Michigan University. Taking this course would already fulfill a Michigan State University requirement. Lynn patiently explained that since I would likely teach multiply impaired children, the Pied Piper experience would be advantageous. Parental jackhammering finally broke down my resistance. This teacher aide position involved creating lesson plans for four students involving (1) identifying colors, (2) handwriting skills, (3) making change, and (4) social skills including table manners and eating techniques to all of them. I enjoyed that very much, including picnics, field trips to Dinosaur Gardens and to Central Michigan University where we observed developmentally disabled children in a learning lab, toured Central Michigan University, and lunched at a fancy restaurant.

The Neil Armstrong Apollo 11, Saturn V Moon Landing occurred July 20, 1969, the night we stayed at Kellogg Center with Mother and Dad prior to MSU orientation. This event will remain memorable indeed as history in the making for both U.S. space exploration and a new life direction for us.

On July 21-22, Nancy and I attended orientation at Michigan State University where we gained experience of staying overnight in a college dorm, selecting our fall courses from the college catalog, and reviewing our selections with an academic advisor. To our delight, we had received our housing assignment to Yakeley Hall several months before. Upon entering MSU in the fall, each of us would be assigned academic advisors for our specific programs of study. Following orientation, I could hardly wait until the fall term opening of Michigan State. Finally, Nancy and I crossed the threshold into an adult world.

CHAPTER 7: AN IRONIC DIRECTION

For many years, I had reacted ambivalently toward autumn until God's spiritual and emotional healing. On one hand, I reveled in its magnificent gold, rust, orange, brown, and scarlet murals against a bright blue sky and in pleasant childhood memories of new clothes, books, school supplies, friends, and teachers when September heralded in each school year. On the other hand, associating late autumn's fallen leaves with an unfulfilled life-long dream triggered sadness.

My desire to teach blind and visually impaired children blossomed through major childhood events. One involved observing a teacher who inspired me during a visit to the Michigan School for the Blind in Lansing, Michigan, already mentioned in Chapter 3. Being inquisitive, I aspired to enchant pupils with life-long discovery learning. Admiring Louis Braille's, Anne Sullivan's, and my teachers' dedication, I strove to follow in their footsteps.

Crystalizing my vocational goal occurred during an eighth-grade field trip to various Lansing points of interest, including the state legislature and Michigan State University. Seeing its huge, sprawling campus consisting of red-bricked buildings including ivy-covered dormitories and rolling, lush, grassy landscapes with an abundance of shrubs, lilacs, and geraniums planted around the buildings, attracted me to enrolling in its special education program. In fact, high school, and Alpena Community College instructors both marveled and quipped, "What a big university for a little girl who doesn't see well!"

During the first month at Michigan State, I eventually located all my classes through trial and error. With Nancy majoring in business education and other dorm mates, I survived the nightly panty raids by the college guys descending on Yakeley Hall, nicknamed "The Convent." I maintained a solid B- average in my classes, enjoyed being on my own, and attended jazz, folk, and classical music concerts.

However, my complacency sharply nosedived one day around the end of October when my academic adviser, Dr. David Munson (fictitious name), abruptly summoned me into his office following a low-vision seminar he conducted.

Assigned to him at the beginning of the term, I had been reassured that since he, too, was blind, he would be a good fit. Yet entering his office that morning filled me with foreboding.

"Sit down. We must talk about your future."

Dr. Munson erectly sat in a high-backed, black leather chair. He impressed me as a distinguished man in his fifties with shocking gray hair. He wore an impeccably pressed charcoal gray and white tweed business suit, white shirt, matching gray tie, socks, and black dress shoes.

"Miss Fortier, I commend you for your academic standing in high school, at Alpena Community College, and so far at Michigan State. However, I foresee two obstacles in teaching which are your visual impairment and your speech. You speak monotonously and so slowly that you could lose attention of the class. Regular elementary teacher certification is required before specialization in teaching the blind."

Suddenly, I felt as if he had punched me in the stomach. What did he mean by impaired vision being a barrier to teaching blind children? Absurd!

"Dr. Munson," I asserted after composing myself, "I do not regard my limited vision as a liability but as an asset. Knowing what having limited vision is like, I can empathize more with visually impaired children than I could if I were fully sighted. Who do you recommend on campus to help me improve my speech?"

Upon Dr. Munson's recommendation, I enrolled in speech therapy three times a week for a whole year at Michigan State University Speech and Audiology Clinic. Even by the end of three months, other professors, family, and friends already noticed a vast improvement in my varied inflections and voice rate. Yet, somehow, Dr. Munson still doubted my ability to teach as his comments implied, "Don't put your eggs too much in one basket. Explore different vocational options."

Raised among former teachers, family and friends who have nurtured within me a positive attitude, I could never understand why Dr. Munson, being blind himself and advising prospective teachers of the blind, viewed blindness or any other physical impairments so negatively. Since he was the only advisor on the MSU faculty for students majoring in special education of the blind and visually impaired, I could not switch to another advisor. Unwilling to transfer to another college, I stuck it out with my parents' encouragement. "Perhaps, Sandy, Dr. Munson is just trying you out right now to see what you are really made of."

From January 10 to May 23, 1970, I volunteered as an aide in the Saturday recreational program at the Michigan School for the Blind to determine whether teaching blind children would be feasible for me. Responsibilities included overseeing bowling, setting pins, distributing roller skates, and playing a modified beeper dodge ball game in gym under Neils Bullock's supervision. At the end of the term, he had given me an excellent evaluation. Realizing that I was not so easily dissuaded from pursuing my vocational goal, Dr. Munson gradually backed off.

From January 4 to March 19, 1971, I student taught in Mrs. Margaret Mendus' first grade class at Pleasant Valley Elementary School, located in New Troy, Michigan, while Nancy student taught at River Valley High School in nearby Three Oaks. The object was teaching in an environment totally different from one's hometown. New Troy, a rural town close to the Michigan/Indiana border, only measured three city blocks and consisted of a post office, an abandoned flour mill, a tavern which a tornado could easily knock over in seconds flat, wooden framed houses with sun porches, two mom-and-pop convenience stores, an elementary, a middle school, and a grill playing 1950s music and closing at 5:00 p.m. The town itself appeared locked into a time warp. As they had done for previous generations, most students still married after graduating from high school and simply remained there for the rest of their lives.

Insisting on staying together, Nancy and I rented a room from Amelia Dinges on Glendora Road in a warm, cozy, little, white house with a sun porch, sandwiched between a little grocery store and a warehouse the size of a small garage. She always made pancakes for breakfast and delicious dinners and desserts, including a favorite with graham cracker crust, cream cheese, cherry or blueberry pie filling, and Cool Whip.

After unpacking, settling in our room, and planning some teaching strategies with the games created in methods courses to add more interest and fun to lessons, how I looked forward to trying them out in class! However, I was forbidden to use these teaching aids since they did not conform to the school district's curriculum. Therefore, I felt thwarted when warned, "Don't be too game happy," and that both the supervising teacher and I would find ourselves in trouble if the visiting superintendent observed something that did not exactly follow the textbook lesson plan. I found teaching these lessons as dull as preparing Hamburger Helper meals without adding any dash of creativity.

In January, Mrs. Mendus asked me to tutor reading to two slow learners, one of whom had recurrent infestations of head lice. Naturally, I did not want to be around her, but I had no choice. Somehow, I managed to move halfway through Book I of *Dick and Jane*, using flashcards printed in different brightly colored felt pens to help these two children distinguish vowels, consonants, and word families from each other.

In February, much to my dismay, teaching became more difficult for me than I had anticipated. Though I could work very well with individuals and small groups, I was extremely nervous teaching the whole class, coupled with the added stress of knowing that my supervising teacher, the student teaching coordinator, and two caseworkers from Services for the Blind were sitting in the back of the classroom observing me. Unable to recognize faces, I could not control the children unless I was standing by their desks. I spoke to the children on an adult level instead of their own. Science lessons especially ended up in disaster like one demonstration in which my lima bean seeds failed to grow into plants because I had placed them in too shallow ground and watered them too much. During another lesson on the earth's rotation, my model of a lamp and a ball representing the sun and the earth rotating on its axis crashed to the floor in smithereens, because I had placed it too close to the edge of my desk. By March 19, all these observers concurred that I needed another term of student teaching. Feeling like the Prodigal Son, I dreaded returning home to tell my parents that I did not do well in student teaching.

It was as unpleasant as I had anticipated. Shaking her head, Mother badgered, "But you wanted to teach since you were yay high. I always thought you loved children."

"You weren't nervous five years ago when those teachers taking that Introduction to Exceptional Children course invited you to give a presentation on blindness at Alpena Community College. People complimented you on it. What has gotten into you now?" she scolded.

Dad spiritedly spoke up in my defense. "Virginia, this is a different ballgame. These were adults! How could you teach a bunch of first graders popping out of their seats every minute like jacks in boxes, running around the room throwing spitballs, and shooting paper wads?"

"Sandy," Mother warned, "Don't mention this to the relatives." Wringing her hands, she cried, "What are you going to do?" Mother had never doubted for a moment that Nancy and I would graduate from college into fulfilling, lucrative careers. Now my future hung in the balance.

Returning that spring to Michigan State University campus to complete other courses required for my B.A. degree, I was scheduled to appear on Monday, April 19, before a committee who would determine whether to allow me a second chance at student teaching after they had heard my case. With a pounding heart, clammy hands, and a dry mouth, I sat at the head of the table, facing seven pairs of penetrating eyes and a volley of questions:

"Miss Fortier, why did you choose teaching as a vocation and who were your teaching models?"

"Why did you decide to attend MSU?"

"How do you feel about working with children?"

Answers to these questions briefly summarized the first three paragraphs of this chapter. Oh! To be anywhere else right then! My head spun so fast I was afraid I would faint. The room closed in on me! When would this ordeal ever end?

"You appear to be a gentle person. How did you control the class?"

"I could control the class while I stood by each student's desk. As the Services for the Blind visitors suggested, my supervising teacher and I made tags in big letters pasted on the chairs so I could see the student's names to help me better discipline them. I also yelled 'Freeze!' to attract their attention."

"What experience did you have working with children before student teaching?"

"From September 8-12, 1969, I observed elementary grade classes at Bingham and McPhee Schools in Alpena, Michigan during a September Experience program offered by MSU and required for prospective elementary teachers."

I also mentioned my summer of 1969 experiences at Pied Piper and volunteering in the Saturday recreation at the Michigan School for the Blind during the second half of my junior year at Michigan State.

"Do you have anything else you would like to say?" Overwhelmed with nervous exhaustion, I paused to collect my thoughts.

"Go on!" someone impatiently urged. "We have another meeting in 40 minutes!"

"Returning to MSU campus, I volunteered as a teacher aide in Mrs. Jean Berkoff's second grade class at Pleasant View Elementary School. There I taught a lesson on safety geared to children's level. This included review questions following a film on strangers. 'What is a stranger?' 'Why am I a stranger?' 'What do you do when a stranger comes up to you and offers you a ride or candy?'"

"During a practicum for course ED 430, Provision for Learning Disabilities, I also volunteered as a teacher aide at Waverly Learning Center. Responsibilities involved assisting learning disabled children with memorizing addition, subtraction, multiplication, and division tables, using blocks and Cuisenaire Rods as instructional materials and M&M's as rewards. I also printed and wrote spelling words in different colored felt pens, cut letters forming words from construction paper or cloth as tactile learning media, and traced letters in the air as a kinesthetic learning approach."

"Given a second chance at student teaching, I would offer the children every educational advantage as I had attempted in the above situations."

Though I believe I had presented a convincing case, it apparently fell on deaf ears. After I returned home from a three-day teaching practicum in Livonia, Michigan on April 28, Mrs. Stauffer, my dorm housemother, met me at the door and ushered me into her office, breaking the news.

"Sandy, I received a telephone call and a letter this week from the MSU board denying you the second term of student teaching. While you were gone, Nancy spoke with the dean of education on your behalf, but I don't know right now whether that will reverse the board's decision."

I sobbed so hard I couldn't stop! She hugged me very tightly and consoled me, "I've made an appointment for you to see Dr. Goodrich at 9:00 tomorrow morning at the counseling center. He will give you a battery of tests to find out what aptitudes you do have and help you determine if teaching or some other vocational goal is really suitable for you."

As Mrs. Stauffer had recommended, I took the vocational interest tests the next day, unsure of what the future would hold for me in teaching. To my astonishment, I scored highest in interests and aptitudes relating to secretarial/office administration, journalism, and law but lowest in scientific, social work, and teaching careers! When Dr. Goodrich advised me to consider secretarial/office administration, I exclaimed, "What! I got C's and D's in high school typing, because holding material up so close to my eyes tremendously slowed down my speed in timed tests. Now you're telling me I qualify for secretarial work?" Dr. Goodrich adamantly reassured me, "Sandy, you'll see! Someday science will invent such things as talking typewriters and calculators, which will open new vistas for the visually impaired in the secretarial field."

Dwelling so much in 1971 on the desolation of a broken dream symbolized by autumn's falling leaves, had I almost ignored God's snapping fingers beckoning me toward a potentially more fulfilling vocation? Would I someday thank Dr. Munson for his role in this? Answers to these probing questions remained to be seen.

CHAPTER 8: NO ROYAL RUNWAY LANDING

Like an inexperienced pilot charting a course, I flew into strong winds, collided into power lines, and nose-dived into rivers instead of taxiing smoothly along the runway toward that dream job at the Michigan Commission for the Blind Training Center. During the summer of 1971, for instance, I took a Michigan civil service examination for a Human Service entry-level position, hoping to obtain employment upon graduation from Michigan State University in December. Since I did not pass, however, I retook it during the fall, but failed again.

That summer, I also wrote to Senator Robert Davis, a Michigan state senator, for his assistance in seeking employment. Following Senator Davis' notification, the Pinconning Public Schools superintendent called me to schedule an interview on Wednesday, September 15, that merely led me into a disappointingly blind alley. Unable to obtain certification, I did not qualify for the teaching positions that were available.

During the afternoons when I had no classes at Michigan State, I applied at employment agencies, such as Kelley Services and Snelling and Snelling, and did cold canvassing at several hotels, but without success. Naively grasping at straws, but undaunted, I even wrote to the draft board in Alpena, Michigan, informing them that I was considering a career in the service and requesting their assistance in finding a niche in a non-combat unit.

Shortly before Christmas while I was upstairs practicing timed typing writings for potential civil service exams, the telephone rang, and Mother answered. Suddenly, she shrieked, "What is going on? Sandy, come downstairs this minute! The sergeant from the local draft board wants to speak to you!"

After he explained that a visual acuity of only 20/80 or above would qualify me for military service, I reassured Mom, "Don't worry. I can't go because he says my visual acuity is too low." Then he chuckled, "You have guts! Able-bodied men would flee to Canada to avoid the draft. Perhaps you may want to consider volunteering for the Peace Corps instead." After I told Dad what I did, he, too, reacted with a welter of astonishment, pride, humor, and relief, "You little scrapper!"

After Christmas, I also relentlessly pursued employment. Mr. Fred Richmond, a new rehabilitation counselor for the Alpena area, encouraged me to develop my own job leads. Heeding his advice, I applied for a secretarial position at the Alpena County Courthouse and as a ward clerk at Alpena General Hospital. During that interview, a nurse counseled me to obtain training in courses to see whether I would enjoy working in an office or in medical transcription. I even applied for substitute teaching openings at the Alpena Public Schools. However, due to the surplus of teachers my age seeking employment, certified teachers already had filled those openings. As time went on, I became discouraged by employers telling me, "We don't know what we can find for a visually impaired person to do," or "We'd love to have you but worry about liability if you fell and injured yourself while walking through the office or plant." Having written to the Alpena Lions Club, I heard nothing from them until one night in October, 1972, when two members soliciting donations showed up at our home. Answering the door, Mother exploded, "How dare you come around collecting when my visually handicapped daughter wrote to you for help in finding employment and received no answer!"

Early in February, 1972, I read an ad in the Alpena News about a consumer forum which Representative Philip Ruppe would conduct at the Alpena Civic Center on Tuesday, February 8. Mother suggested talking to him. After listening intently and sympathetically to my concerns, he promised to do whatever he could to help me.

As an alumna of Alpena Community College, I also sought job placement services there. When the employment placement specialist barked, "Tell me about yourself," I began reciting my resumé verbatim. Suddenly he ranted, "I can read your resumé! How does your education and past employment such as summer jobs relate to the positions you are seeking?" Then, for me, that was difficult to answer spontaneously. "Why don't you look directly at me when I talk to you?" the placement specialist demanded. I explained, "That's the way my eyes function. Due to retinopathy at premature birth, I lack central vision and can only see peripherally, not directly."

"I don't give a damn how your eyes function!" he snapped. "To me, as an employer, your lack of eye contact reveals that you are trying to hide something." By this time, intimidation set in. Was this a psychological ploy to ascertain how I would deal with a ticking-time-bomb-boss?

This last comment totally flummoxed me, "Your grades are too good. You should have been out drinking and raising hell while in college." Oh, to have zinged him with this comeback, "How I'd love to have thrown a late-night beer party with stereo blasting right in your front yard!"

Depending upon my mood, today I either would have angrily told him to go to Holy Hannah or have asserted, "I don't understand why you're so angry. I wish you could treat me as respectfully as you would like to be treated." If his sarcasm continued, I would have left. Yet, to his credit, the placement specialist did give me some hints on answering open-ended questions. So, I bungled the interview but could chalk it up to a valuable learning experience.

In the meantime, Nancy who was working for Arthur Andersen & Co. accounting firm in Detroit, contacted Mr. Benjamin Pumo and Anthony Tamer, Placement Specialist of Goodwill Industries, combined with the Detroit League for the Handicapped. Then I wrote to them setting up appointments on Thursday, March 30, 1972.

I remember Detroit Goodwill/League for the Handicapped as a huge, red-bricked building but nothing about the inside. After completing applications for services from Mr. Tamer, I talked with Mr. Pumo who stated that I was overqualified to work in a Goodwill agency, and that it did not offer a substantial training program, adding that Goodwill would pay by piecework. He also voiced the opinion that to be employed, I would have to mature more. I should have asked him what he meant by "mature". Fred Richmond, my case worker, teased, "Who wants to mature? It simply means that you're getting old!"

Returning home, I also completed applications through the Michigan Employment Security Commission and Reitz and LaFleche, CPAs' for employment. Handing me an accounting ledger, Mr. LaFleche asked if I could see well enough to fill out one of those. Straining to see the lines, I woefully admitted I would be fooling nobody but myself. Again, I contacted Representative Philip Ruppe regarding difficulty seeking employment. Like a dog nipping at heels of sheep straying from the flock, he contacted Services for the Blind, demanding "What are you doing for Sandra Fortier?"

One afternoon, Mr. David Search, a rehabilitation teacher, arrived at our house to discuss the vending stand program with me. However, considering the precariousness of owning any business, I was not interested in pursuing employment as a vending stand operator.

Plagued with such a low self-esteem during this time, I could not advocate for myself. Overhearing the phrase "vending stand operator" while painting the inside of kitchen cupboards, Mother jumped from the ladder, flew into the living room, and yelled, "How about selling pencils on street corners? She's too intelligent for that!" He then advised me to consider Dictaphone transcription.

Shortly thereafter, I received information from Services for the Blind regarding a nine-month medical transcription program offered through the Chicago Lighthouse for the Blind and another course offered from June 26 to August 4, 1972 for blind adults at the Michigan School for the Blind. Unfamiliar with Chicago, I had many qualms, because attending the Lighthouse required finding an off-campus room or apartment. Although mobility instructors from the Lighthouse would travel with me on the Chicago "L" to classes for two weeks, after that, they would expect me to travel back and forth independently. This would be daunting, in-

deed, for someone from a small town like Alpena. Within a day or two, Mr. Richmond telephoned me regarding
my decision. I opted for the on-campus Michigan School
for the Blind medical transcription program, which he
affirmed was a wise decision.

On June 25, Mother and Dad drove me to MSB and
settled me in an assigned Longhouse E dorm room. I
am grateful to those house parents who allowed me to
stay in the dorm on weekends as it enabled me to save
money otherwise used for bus transportation home or
staying in Lansing motels.

The medical transcription class consisted of eight
students ranging in age from 18 to 45 with Mr. Dickerson, our teacher. Each day, students typed or Brailled
spelling lists of medical terms pertaining to a particular
branch of medicine and their meaning as Mr. Dickerson
dictated them for later study as homework. The next day
the class transcribed medical reports from Dictaphone
belts containing these words. I kept up with the taped
dictation even as it increased to 80 w.p.m. though the
average speed was about 55 w.p.m.! My lost self-confidence revived! After dinner, my roommate and I quizzed
each other on the terms. Then I joined other students in
on-campus fun consisting of swimming, bowling, talent
shows, and hootenannies.

Teaching eating techniques to the blind has revolu-
tionized since my parents and I visited MSB in 1954. Volunteering as a weekend houseparent aide during that
summer I took medical transcription, I observed children eating on regular plates.

After completing the medical transcription course, I
found a welcome respite from job hunting when traveling to Quebec and Toronto, Canada, strolling down
Old Quebec's quaint, narrow cobblestone streets, and
savoring crepes. So devoted to Mary, the Blessed Mother
of Jesus, and knowing that people visiting the Shrine of
Sainte-Anne-de-Beaupré had received miraculous cures
for physical afflictions, we, therefore, believed that by
visiting that shrine, Ste. Anne, the mother of Mary, too,
would guide me in finding employment.

To my initial disappointment, the distant Sainte-Anne-
de-Beaupré mosaics and stained-glass windows in its Ba-
silica vault appeared to me as nondescript blobby shapes

and colors like a child's collage consisting of construction paper, plastic, or felt pasted on a wooden board. However, the subsequent guidance of Sainte Anne and My Mother of Perpetual Help shining as a beacon to me throughout job hunting and the rest of my life would prove more luminous than the visual appearance of the shrine. The awareness of Mary's miraculous birth to Sainte Anne and Joachim despite their barrenness during their first 20 years of marriage finally renewed my hope of eventually finding employment. The discarded crutches (from miracles) mounted in the church rafters poignantly affirmed that light would appear at the end of this emotional tunnel to a fulfilling role in life even though it might require more time for me than for someone else. How swiftly the serenity and faith yearned for so long enveloped me there!

The Canada vacation psychologically fueled another employment search in anticipation of a smoother landing. This included meeting Mr. Kench, a tall, lanky, red-haired, bespectacled placement specialist from Grand Rapids. Soon, telephone calls from Detroit, Gaylord, Grand Rapids, and Ann Arbor regarding medical transcription openings deluged. However, these available openings only specified working afternoon and evening shifts which aroused many misgivings of living in a location which required catching two to three buses or taxicabs to and from work alone at night. As Dad teased, "The $1.75-$2.50 hourly wages offered would barely earn enough to buy the leggings of a hummingbird, let alone sufficiently cover room or apartment rent, utilities, groceries, and transportation expenses." Though placement specialists threatened to discontinue sponsorship through Services for the Blind for further training or financial assistance if I refused employment, I stood my ground against accepting any job that would jeopardize my safety or chances of advancement.

Hoping that I could obtain some low vision magnifiers that would help me read printed copies without holding them so close to my eyes when taking timed writings on employment typing tests, Fred Richmond, my case worker, scheduled me for a low vision appointment for Monday, October 16 with Dr. Morris Mintz at Mt. Sinai Hospital in Detroit which proved futile. Though monocular magnifiers allowed me to read the entire eye charts, I could only read beginnings and ends of printed words but nothing in the middle. Puzzled, Dr. Mintz theorized that since people see with their minds as well as their eyes, my mind apparently fills in what my eyes miss in reading print.

Mother purchased a copy of Harold Krents' book *To Race the Wind* as a Christmas present to motivate me. I do not remember exactly where she bought it. Mother and I had previously heard about Harold Krents during a televised November 24, 1968 panel discussion featuring him and three other blind college students on the David Susskind Show. Harold impressed us as being brilliant, articulate, and humorous in expressing his aspirations to become a lawyer and his reactions to public prejudice toward blindness.

He inspired me as a hero to whom I could relate in many respects. Like me, he was born in the late 1940s with retinopathy at prematurity and grew up in the 1950s through 1960s. Our parents advocated for mainstreaming in regular classes. In elementary school, he and I contended with stern teachers and bullying classmates. Naturally, I identified with Harold's adolescent loneliness and his difficulty in seeking employment within law firms. His warmth and wit radiate throughout his autobiography. Reading about Harold's tenacity eventually jumpstarted mine in seeking employment.

In the meantime, going nowhere with the employment search, I decided to enroll in an office procedures course at Alpena Community College. During this time, I took and passed a federal civil service examination with an average score of 85%, excelling in verbal more than in quantitative reasoning.

A cousin suggested praying to St. Jude, patron saint of the impossible, for help in securing employment. Mother and I also steadfastly attended Thursday night rosary services at St. Mary's church, as well as Lenten Friday evening Stations of the Cross at St. John the Baptist Church in Alpena for this intention.

On April 24, 1973, two days after Easter, Mr. Richmond arrived, notifying us that a state civil service vacancy for a typist-clerk occurred at the Michigan Rehabilitation Center for the Blind on Oakland Drive in Kalamazoo. It entailed filing, transcribing Center rehabilitation teachers', counselors', and consulting psychologist's reports from dictation belts, answering the telephone, relaying messages to a supervising counselor and later composing letters and memos for a supervising counselor. After he asked if I would be interested, I jubilantly hollered, "Yes!" After he left, I immediately typed and sent a letter with accompanying résumé notifying Mr. Louis Martin, then Program Manager, of my interest in the position. A month before I had already applied to Michigan Department of Civil Service for the six-months' appointment on a trial basis in lieu of taking the exam as an employment accommodation for people with disabilities.

To avoid making the same mistakes in previous interviews, I strategically planned some answers to anticipated questions the Center staff might ask. For example, to "Tell me about yourself," I would indicate that by being visually impaired, I could empathize with the blind students and staff. I also planned to highlight my conscientiousness, eagerness to learn, filing experience at the Hinks School and Alpena Community College Libraries and knowledge of medical and psychological terms as an asset in typing counseling reports. Asked to name one of my weaknesses, I would admit to nervousness and self-consciousness, but add that gaining on-the-job experience would overcome both. I also made a kit consisting of typing paper, correction tape, and eraser should I be required to demonstrate my typing skills.

On Monday, April 30, Mr. Louis Martin from the Michigan Rehabilitation Center for the Blind telephoned and scheduled me for an interview at 11:00 on Wednesday, May 2.

When my parents and I arrived at the Center, Mr. Martin introduced me to Kathryn Pavey, Account Clerk, and Alice Kisen, secretary to Mr. Robert Wisner, the Center director. Then he reiterated what he had spoken during my telephone interview about the job and that he was impressed with my neatly typed letter and résumé. I remarked about the manicured grounds, the peacefulness of the residential area surrounding the building, and how the Center would be a very pleasant place to work.

Betty Jacobs, Director of Diagnostic Services, more intensely interviewed me. Having anticipated interview questions landed a home run, because she asked me to tell her about the relevancy of my college courses as well as strengths to the typist-clerk position. How impressed she was with my foresight of bringing the kit of typing paper, typing eraser, and correction tape though the Center furnished these supplies! To verify my typing ability, she instructed me to transcribe a dictated counseling final report, a letter, a memo, and an authorization. Though she expected some mistakes since I was typing on an unfamiliar Selectric, overall, Betty was pleased with the documents I transcribed from Dictaphone.

In the morning, I took the Center tour, including industrial arts, orientation and mobility, cooking, and oral-aural communications classes. Towards afternoon, Mr. Robert Wisner, Director, ushered my parents and me into his conference room. "Sandy, you have the job! When would you be willing to start?"

"I'd begin next week in a heartbeat if I didn't have two Alpena Community College clerical courses to finish. I'm like a filly ready for the race!"

"Since you have only two weeks left, you complete those courses! How about beginning on May 21?" I agreed though I could hardly wait to begin work.

After Mr. Wisner informed us that I had the job, tears rolled down Mother's cheeks. No longer her baby, soon I would be flying away from the nest for good. Patting her on the shoulder, Mr. Wisner reassured her, "Don't cry! Sandy will do fine. Besides, I am married to a woman who is also blind." Returning home, I wrote a thank you note to the staff for the interview and the position. At last, happy landing on the job tarmac, thanks to the intercession of St. Jude, St. Anne, and the Blessed Virgin Mary!

CHAPTER 9: EYE OPENERS

The weekend I arrived in Kalamazoo, I still pinched myself. Finally, in two days, I would start employment at the Michigan Rehabilitation Center for the Blind and be self-supporting. No more badgering from well-meaning, concerned, but nosy relatives and friends, "Do you have a job yet?"

I was ready to conquer the world, including a six months' backlog of dictated but not transcribed reports left by the previous typist who regretfully went blind due to a severe undiagnosed eye infection. Ah! Many lessons to learn and new experiences to savor from now until retirement! I could hardly wait to begin!

Before I could even think of tackling that backlog of transcription awaiting me, my orientation began with mandatory immersion training as a blind student. I was shocked to discover how much I had functioned visually despite my retinopathy of prematurity. Suddenly plunged into darkness and disoriented in space and time terrified me. In fact, walking under the blindfold with a sighted guide from my office to the bus stop seemed like an eternity. Throughout the day I dusted furniture, made a grilled cheese sandwich, and sliced a cucumber under the occlude or blindfold (Miraculously, my fingers were still intact!). While completing these tasks, I wore glasses simulating various visual impairments of glaucoma, diabetic retinopathy, retinal detachment, tunnel vision, and cataracts. This activity fulfilled its purpose of developing empathy needed to interact with newly blinded persons.

The next day I discovered an interesting history regarding services for the blind in Michigan. During the first part of the twentieth century, services for the blind consisted of a sheltered workshop in Saginaw and the blind concession program. In the 1950s, the Michigan Department of Social Services (DSS) assigned a few case-workers to a Blind Only caseload to provide financial and employment assistance. A few years later, the DSS combined the workshop, blind concessions, and these caseworkers into a Division of Services for the Blind.

In the mid-1960s, a group of state legislators recog-nized that the broom-making workshop in Saginaw pre-sented a demeaning image of blind workers and should be closed. After studying other state programs, they de-cided that a new facility should be constructed empha-sizing independence rather than sheltered work. There-fore, the Center now known as the Bureau of Services for Blind Persons Training Center has operated since 1970.

I must mention that during my employment, the Cen-ter had been known by two other names. Initially it was called the Michigan Rehabilitation Center for the Blind until October 1, 1978, when the governor appointed a five-member commission to represent blind consumers and to oversee services provided by the renamed Mich-igan Commission for the Blind Training Center. There-fore, I refer to it by these names as well as "MCBTC" or "the Center" in my book. It has offered a residential, comprehensive program of personal adjustment train-ing and vocational exploration.

JOB AND LIFE LESSONS

The first six months of probation subjected me to an overwhelming blur of new names, policies, innumerable procedures, and tremendous stress due to my fear of failure following that student teaching debacle. Again, thanks to God, family, and staff support, I survived. My probation ending on November 16, 1973, gave me a lot to celebrate at Thanksgiving. Finally, a permanent civil service employee! Hurray!

Transcribing Reports

Transcribing reports revealed interesting stories about each student while affording me the opportunity to learn about daily living skills the Center taught to the blind. These involved personal management skills including grooming, laundry, identifying clothing styles and colors with clothing tags, and identifying paper money by folding denominations in different ways, talking and Braille clocks. Handwriting covered signature guides as well as letter formation. Low-vision class dealt with magnifiers such as monocular, hand, and close circuit TV magnifiers. Oral-aural Communications introduced me to different types of recorders, reading, and talking book machines. Occupational Therapy and counseling reports I transcribed helped me to recognize the students as people, not merely clients or numbers. Like teachers and counselors, I had to guard against prejudice.

Being a gourmand, I especially enjoyed transcribing adaptive kitchen skills training reports since I could discover what students were baking or cooking.

I did complete my inherited six-month backlog of transcription in three months. Each day, I persevered, but combined fun with work by challenging myself to beat my own record. This approach helped me to relax.

Initially, I transcribed material from a Lanier Business Products belt transcriber and thereafter switched to transcribing from a General Electric Modified Cassette Recorder, because the staff could dictate more on cassettes than they could on belts.

Advantages of Adaptive Technology

Proud of having been the only visually impaired student mainstreamed into the Alpena Public Schools without low-vision devices and ashamed of my limited vision, I initially resisted using adaptive equipment to aid in transcribing and typing authorizations, such as the Apollo close circuit television, which resembled an ordinary television set with a camera mounted over the typewriter. I sat hunched over the typewriter until a stiff neck, tired eyes, and Betty Jacobs' persuasion finally convinced me that using this device would improve typing efficiency and proofreading accuracy.

Employee Insights Regarding Difficulty in Transferring Calls

Now, I recognize how mental circuits overload, but as a new employee, I blamed mistakes on stupidity rather than on unfamiliarity with office procedures and attempts to absorb everything all at once. To my chagrin and frustration, for instance, I initially had difficulty transferring calls. In 1973, transferring calls under our Centrex system to the receptionist required pushing a small metal transfer lever under the receiver cradle down and up, which was very tricky since pressing that metal lever too lightly would not transfer the call and pressing it too hard disconnected the call. Once the call was transferred, the receptionist routed it from her switchboard to the appropriate person in the building. Perhaps being left alone with the Bell Telephone Company representative instructing me at my own pace, I would have mastered this procedure better than with Betty Jacobs hovering and interrupting, "Do you understand this? Or is it still clear as mud?" Though Betty did show genuine concern, her nervous fluttering around like a red-headed magpie distracted and annoyed me. Yet, being a new employee, I hesitated to tell her this. Years later to my relief, telephones which operated by dialing the in-house staff to notify them of incoming calls, pressing a pause switch, and then pressing a conference call button to connect the outside callers to staff persons receiving calls enabled me to transfer calls more easily.

Lessons from Staff

Suzanne Johnson, a transplant from Tennessee and a blind rehabilitation teacher working at the Center from 1971 through 1976, befriended me. During my first few lonely months at work, she invited me for lunch at a Servateen in the Kalamazoo State Hospital run by Jerry Francisco, a blind vendor. Seeing how successful and confident he was also uplifted me. She always included me when she invited the staff over to dinner and sincerely appreciated my work.

Besides her compassion and encouragement, I admired her assertive and down-to-earth personality presented in her teaching reports, spontaneous expression of her opinions at staff meetings, and unconcern at what married people thought about her singleness. Regretfully, we lost touch when she left the Center.

I also owe tremendous appreciation to other teachers and counselors for rescuing me from the mire of unfamiliar terminology, particularly the Industrial Arts teacher who patiently explained that the correct term in a report was "wood screws" not "work screws" and that a "plumber's snake" and a "plumber's friend" both functioned in clearing drains. Through helpful explanations, I eventually absorbed the industrial arts, counseling, and occupational therapy lingo characteristic of educational progress reports.

Betty Lujan-Roberts for whom I transcribed many Braille educational reports introduced me to a Braille slate and stylus and braille numbers. Walking by her classes, I noticed how she passionately taught Braille. She enjoyed cracking jokes and Center activities. Her personality spiced up our days like salsa on a burrito.

Having attended regular classes and stable vision, I never learned Braille. How blind people can read Braille mystified me since I had difficulty distinguishing the dots with my fingertips.

These teachers also reinforced an indelible lesson regarding the hazards of traveling without a white cane during my third week on the job following a hair-raising incident of almost being hit while crossing a street. Until then, I never traveled with a white cane in Alpena because people there knowing my limited vision had always stopped to let me cross. On a cloudy day, I can more easily distinguish white and orange "Walk/Don't Walk" sign lights than I can on a sunny day when the incident occurred. By the grace of God, a motorist just missed hitting me.

The next day, all the Center staff who had witnessed the whole incident greeted me as I entered the front door, "From now on, you're carrying a white cane for identification!"

"No, I'm not!" I protested. "People will think I'm totally blind."

"Better for them to know you are blind than to run you over. Legally, if you were injured because of not carrying the white cane for identification, you may lose your case in court," they warned.

Larry King, an orientation and mobility instructor, showed me how to grip and arc the cane by swinging it from side to side, and to listen for parallel traffic on my right, left, and in front of me, guiding me when to stop and to cross streets as a supplement to visually identifying landmarks, curbs, and drop-offs. From then on, I have always traveled more confidently with a cane.

Partially sighted like me, my first supervisor, Betty Jacobs, rode on every bus route with me to familiarize me with the Kalamazoo Metro Bus system and instructed me on making time calls to Yellow Cab, specifying the date, time, pick-up location, and destination. Unlike larger cities such as Detroit or New York where people hailed cabs, in Kalamazoo, people summoned cabs by making time calls.

Lessons from Cab Drivers

The taxi drivers presented a motley cast of interesting characters. Affable Sherman Rose, for example, acquired a phenomenal memory for locations and directions and a fascinating hobby of learning new words in foreign languages which he tried to teach me but without success. Another driver and his visiting cousin helped me get rid of a neighbor's cat that sneaked into my apartment. First, the cousin gently encircled and lured it with a bowl of milk. While the cat drank the milk, the driver then scooped it into his arms, caressed, and carried it out the door. I also learned to avoid persistently flirtatious drivers like downed power lines, only requesting cabbies whom I respected and vice versa.

Lessons from Emma Evarts

Though petite in stature, Emma Evarts with whom I stayed, was gargantuan in wisdom. During the first week in Kalamazoo, Emma walked with me to the Kalamazoo Public Library to obtain my library card and encouraged me to subscribe to the *Kalamazoo Gazette.* "A good citizen is an informed citizen," she insisted and advised me to read inspirational literature instead of wasting time on trash.

One Saturday afternoon, I went to the Kalamazoo County Fair without informing Emma. When I returned, she was upset, because Mother and Dad had called her, and she did not know where I was. Wagging her finger, she scolded, "Remember, the choices you make and the people you meet will shape your destiny!"

As a former history teacher, Emma emphasized discussions on reasons events happened, not memorization of dates, which I would have found more meaningful in school. Not allowing her vision loss due to macular degeneration to deter her from being informed, she avidly listened to televised daily and evening local and national news programs and to talking books from the State of Michigan Library for the Blind and Physically Handicapped. Her discussions of talking books she had read inspired me to read those books. She enjoyed reading mostly nonfiction books, including biographies and autobiographies, as well as fictional books based on fact, such as *Gone with the Wind* and Charles Dickens' classics. Most of all, she loved stimulating political discussions. With maturity, now I value her enjoyment in sharing her knowledge about history and current events. How I wish that I had joined her more often in watching these programs instead of burying myself in my room for hours on end!

I eventually grasped Emma's philosophy regarding choices the hard way after I regretted my impulsiveness in answering a *Kalamazoo Gazette* Jottings ad for membership in a fall ladies' bowling league. Arriving there on the first night, I discovered that Blue Crystal Lanes was in a rundown neighborhood near the fairgrounds. While bowling throughout the evening, I also had misgivings about those other team members, two of whom even I could see physically resembled oversized comic-strip caricatures of Blondie and Betty Boop. The third told crude jokes, swore, and chain-smoked. All three women discussed their frequent encounters with men at bars, potential pitfalls I wanted to avoid. Finally heeding my better judgment, I immediately returned home, and the next day, I notified Blue Crystal Lanes of my withdrawal from the league.

Longing for friendship during the fall of 1973, I also plunged into a young adult prayer group involved with the charismatic Catholic movement begun in 1972. Unnerved by members praying in tongues to the Holy Spirit, I left that group.

Finally learning to choose friends and activities more wisely, I immersed myself into church activities such as singing in choir and contributing to bake sales. Months later, I even had more fun bowling on a Center league at Eastland Bowl than I did at Blue Crystal Lanes.

I also joined the Kalamazoo Community Chorale. Planting the seed, another church choir member also belonging to that group, invited me to their 1978 Christmas concert. Bursting with excitement after the concert, I could hardly wait until January to join the Chorale.

Besides our annual spring and Christmas community concerts, the Chorale sang at nursing homes and the Kalamazoo State Hospital. I reveled in the audience applause and foot tapping to the music and in knowing that my singing, too, brightened these people's lives. I also volunteered to sing in the talent shows following our annual Christmas banquets.

I cannot imagine God giving us this gift of music and not being able to share it with others. What a more glorious opportunity than a Sing for the Cure?

Janet Berghorst, a former director, suggested, "Ladies, for 2001, let's present a Southwestern Michigan Sing. This will replicate the Sing for the Cure premiered in Dallas, Texas on June 11, 2000, celebrating establishment of the Susan G. Komen Breast Cancer Foundation."

"Yes!" we unanimously roared.

However, our enthusiasm suddenly dampened when Jan announced, "All other auditoriums in Kalamazoo are booked solidly until fall, but we do have an opening at Chenery Auditorium at 8:30 p.m. on Friday, April 13."

"Friday, the 13th! You're crazy!" exclaimed a Chorale member raising her eyebrows. "Don't you realize it's Good Friday?"

"With evening services, no one will come," warned the other.

"Quiet!" Jan shouted. "We commemorate our Lord's Passion and death on Good Friday, don't we? Why not also remember those ravaged by cancer? They, too, carry their heavy crosses. Have faith!"

Like Simon of Cyrene, initially we, too, reluctantly helped Jesus represented in those afflicted with cancer to carry His cross but for different reasons. Not knowing who Jesus was, for instance, why should Simon have helped a stranger condemned as a criminal? Likewise, we did not want anything else to interfere with our own traditional Good Friday observances and Easter celebrations. Fortunately, Jan stood her ground; otherwise, we would have missed a potentially blessed opportunity. Especially for me, it meant singing as a tribute to Emma Evarts whom I described earlier in this section. She, herself, succumbed to dying from breast cancer.

From January 8 until April 9, 2001, the SW Michigan Sing for the Cure Chorus comprised of the Kalamazoo Community Chorale, Male Chorus, and church choirs throughout southwestern Michigan, practiced twice a week. Unable to sight read music, I memorized it by listening to a CD of the Dallas, Texas Sing for the Cure in addition to attending rehearsals.

Since the movements of the other members appeared blurry to me, I had difficulty snapping my fingers and clapping in sync with "Living Out Loud Blues" and "Groundless Ground" within the "Taking Control" portions of the piece. Sensing my frustration, a chorus member sitting next to me, coaxed, "You can do it! I'll nudge you when it's time to snap or clap." Before long, I synchronized my movements with those of everyone else.

Finally, the long-anticipated evening arrived! The warm-up room buzzed with excitement while the chorus lined up to process on stage. Imagine being the only chorus to sing the whole Sing for the Cure suite after it was premiered in Texas!

Though intending to maintain a professional demeanor as a "Sing" chorus, we eventually lost our composure when the ominous percussion-piano sledge-hammer prelude and the percussion death-rattle crescendos near the end of "Who Will Speak?" sent shivers down our spines. Yet, "Who Will Speak?" also impressed upon us that, as God had commanded, we acted as our brothers' keepers. In our passionate "Sing for the Cure," we ministered to the ill and suffering with the ardent support of 1,000 people in attendance at Chenery Auditorium to raise money for cancer cures.

As we sang "Borrowed Time" and "The Promise Lives On," tears also welled within us and streamed down our faces.

While the "Sing" progressed, chorus members and the audience reacted more diversely, depending upon their experiences with cancer. During "The Child's Voice—Come to Me, Mother," a black-and-white 1939 scrapbook photo image of Mother's face etched with wistfulness and abandonment shortly after her mother died flashed through my mind. Suddenly, I broke down sobbing! Noticing this, another chorus member whispered, "I know this must be very difficult for you but hang in there." Before long, most of the other women sobbed and hugged each other while singing this piece and "The Mother's Voice—Who Will Curl My Daughter's Hair?" as well. Men furtively dabbed their eyes with soggy handkerchiefs. I could not ascertain the audience's reaction, but according to the *Kalamazoo Gazette* review, one woman in the audience left the auditorium because the piece was too emotional for her.

Dad and I choked up during "The Sister's Voice—Girl in the Mirror" because the inseparable bonding between a woman and her sister who died of cancer reminded us of my sister's and mine as twins. Mother stated how the tapestry prominently displayed in the lobby of Chenery Auditorium including her mother's name inscribed along with 99 other names in it meant so much. Then that tapestry inscribed with more names of remembered cancer victims traveled to other Southwestern Michigan cities where it was displayed in other auditoriums performing Sing for the Cure. What an inspiring legacy to cancer victims and their families!

During "Groundless Ground," our electrified audience's clapping and stomping that filled the room would have even done a religious revival meeting proud!

How I wished Emma Evarts, too, was there in the audience! Yet I imagined her in heaven proudly cheering me on, "Bravo! Way to go!" I passionately sang as a tribute to her and to other cancer victims and survivors.

During the closing, "One Voice—Proclaiming Hope", the lights in the auditorium went out except for the spotlight shining on the two soloists. Then as the chorus sang, little flashlights resembling candles were turned on one by one in each row until all were lit, symbolizing how with one voice we can all make a difference, proclaiming victory, hope, and faith in finding new cancer cures. The chorus received a standing ovation.

Performing the Sing for the Cure harshly reminded us how cancer kills, maims, and blinds. During this concert, my heart ached for people suffering from the ravages of eye and breast cancer, such as countless students at the Michigan Commission for the Blind Training Center.

Southwestern Michigan Sing for the Cure immersed me in a drama involving a cast of real cancer victims, survivors, and their caregivers while it commemorated Jesus' Passion and Resurrection that these victims and survivors symbolized. Therefore, I would describe the Easter of 2001 as the most meaningful and inspirational one I have ever celebrated!

Imagine singing 34 years with the Kalamazoo Community Chorale! We've shared a lot together, happy times and sad ones. I am grateful to have had the chance to enjoy singing beautiful music and many life-long friendships that have enriched my life.

Orientation and Mobility

I have observed orientation and mobility instructors at the Michigan Commission for the Blind Training Center repeating the mantra "No One Eats Soggy Waffles" to aid students in recalling directions as well as demonstrating orientation and mobility techniques of carrying, arcing, and sliding the cane to detect drop-offs and stairs, and listening for parallel traffic to cross streets and intersections. Further prompting to determine position in space, instructors questioned, "If you were facing North, which direction would be if you turned left (or right, or backward)?" Being directionally challenged, myself, I am amazed how totally blind people know where they are. For this reason, I have difficulty grasping the concept of GPS.

On April 20, 1983, our entire MCBTC staff traveled to Leader Dogs for the Blind School at 1039 Rochester Road in Rochester Hills, Michigan. Fund-raising projects garner money needed to provide Leader Dog training programs. Though Leader Dogs for the Blind School offers an accelerated seven-day orientation and mobility program in cane travel, guide dog training, and GPS or Global Positioning System, our tour concentrated on guide dogs. This presentation emphasized the importance of caring for and bonding with the dog during the first three days of the 26-day program; appropriate commands and praise; and tour of the examining room for dogs, the lab, and kennels. We even participated in role play as candidates for dog guide training under the blindfold. Matched with a medium-size black Labrador which really put me through my paces by pulling me while it was in harness, I understood why a trainee must be in excellent physical shape to be accepted into the program. The dorm rooms like those of the Michigan Commission for the Blind Training Center contained a bed, dresser, closet, and bathroom but included platforms for the guide dogs. Circular tables filled the dining room where piping hot meals were served family style. We also rode the bus transporting students and their guide dogs to downtown Rochester where they received mobility lessons and practice.

I was happy for the opportunity to visit the Leader Dogs for the Blind School in Rochester. It gave me a better conception of time and effort involved in orientation and mobility training with a guide dog.

Assuming Other Responsibilities

Besides transferring calls and transcribing reports and correspondence from cassette tape, my job duties involved considerable filing. At first, I was unsure about the rules of filing and needed much support but was motivated to learn and improved. I also filled out service authorizations, which at first entailed typing on multicopy forms regarding psychological, low-vision evaluations through Western Michigan University Low Vision Clinic, and work evaluations through John R. Jenkins Vocational Rehabilitation Center, later changed to Goodwill Industries of S.W. Michigan, in Kalamazoo. Eventually that form was revised to one page that could be corrected with correction tape and later to computerized forms.

Following conversion from our 1987 computer DOS to Windows in 1997, Larry King, my supervisor, suggested I become more proficient in using the mouse by playing computer Solitaire. I must confess I was having so much fun playing Solitaire that I overextended my break. When he entered my office to give me some tapes to transcribe, my face blushed. How I wished there were a hole under my desk to swallow me!

"What have you been doing?" he gravely demanded.

"Practicing mouse skills." I quivered.

"Mouse skills? Mouse skills?" he teased, "Don't let that become habit forming."

Besides computer Solitaire, Larry taught me to laugh at my mistakes by reminding me, "Don't sweat the small stuff. You can't wreck the computer!" If I were glum or preoccupied, he chuckled, "Are you playing the World Serious game today?"

As time went on, duties evolved into typing Student Class Count reports and formulating a procedural manual explaining my responsibilities step by step which enabled coworkers to cover for me while I was ill or on vacation.

Learning from Students

Talking with students, I learned so much from them, because they told their own interesting stories. In fact, one student even taught me some German words! She and I also engaged in a spirited discussion about American parents' attitudes toward students' success contrasted with those in Germany. She stated that German parents emphasize high academic achievement; whereas American parents stress too much importance on popularity and success in sports.

As staff taught students many independent living skills, they, too, learned about students' needs and goals. Transcribing from progress reports helped me do that.

Acquiring Human Sensitivity

Though mastering required skills and keeping abreast of adaptive technology available to the blind daunts any employee, I must admit that learning how to deal with many different personalities proved the most challenging. Uncle Leonard Ruczynski, retired after many years of grocery store ownership/management often advised, "We all have our idiosyncrasies. Remember that when serving customers or clients." To illustrate, reading books, such as Tom Brokaw's *The Greatest Generation* or Tim Russert's *Big Russ and Me*, would have helped me build more rapport with a business manager and an account clerk who grew up during the Depression. As a case in point, I rankled both by flaunting my degree from Michigan State. Presuming to know everything that I needed to know about being a secretary, I requested a promotion after working at the Center for a year.

Gasping with surprise and chuckling, these two veteran employees explained that eligibility for a civil service promotion would depend upon an available opening at the Center or elsewhere, my qualifications, and subsequent application for the position. Naturally, like their contemporaries arduously climbing the career ladder for many years, these coworkers had regarded me as a young upstart. Overhearing the account clerk one day lamenting to someone about how "college graduates lack common sense" stung me like a well-deserved swat across the buttocks. Honestly, looking back, I still had much to learn over several years regarding style formats, transferring calls, and civil service policies. Once I admitted this, the business manager and the account clerk were more willing to teach me. Undoubtedly putting me in my place, God spoke to me through their wisdom as His Son Jesus admonished the apostles James and John against their ambition of being automatically granted the seats to His right and to His left in heaven, described in Mark 10:35-44. In retrospect, I humbly owe my success to these coworkers' grounded advice. Finally, with maturity, respect won over previous dismissal of the business manager and the account clerk as stodgy old fogies.

Gaining Perspective

The most difficult lesson for me as a young adult in my late twenties and early thirties was that Nancy and I as twins did not need to ride the same curling wave throughout life. Wherever that wave carried me, why not always trust it to Jesus? I must confess, I did not. Feeling stigmatized among married friends who called me out on being single or tried to match me with potential partners I disliked, I wondered if I would marry or stay single. To enlighten me, one of Mother's letters walloped me with her wisdom.

"Oh, Sandy, there you go! Worrying again about marriage and what people think. If Jesus wants marriage for you, He'll take care of it. When will you realize that you're an individual in your own right? Marriage or singleness does not make a person. Character does."

Mother continued, "About falling in love, Sandy, I can't answer you on that. I do know that you have things other people do not have and life is not total. You must play the cards with which you are dealt."

"Marriage isn't all that blissful. If I were young in this era, perhaps, I, too, would be single. I know many people are happy being single, and that singleness is meant for them as marriage is meant for others."

Her letter ended, "I, too, wonder what the future has in store for me. At my age, I must cherish good health. We will all face uncertainties, but we cannot become morbid over things. Here is a good philosophy: Yesterday is past, today is within my grasp. Tomorrow is to use or lose for eternity."

I needed that!

Mother's philosophy regarding living in the present moment applied years later when the following events challenged my faith and mettle, trivializing any concerns that had bothered me in my twenties and thirties.

A Hair Raising Ride

Boarding the Greyhound bus from Alpena to Kalamazoo, Michigan on July 10, 1994, after visiting my parents, I noticed an eerie silence punctuated by occasional coughing instead of the usual banter and lively conversations. Politics, recent job promotions, vacations, weddings, and stories about grandchildren had gotten off at the last bus stop. Approaching my seat, I heard two men in two rows behind me laughing at something everyone sensed was rather sinister. Hair stood up on the back of my neck.

Furtively glancing at the men, I discovered that one resembled a caricature of Mr. Clean, sported a mohawk, and wore a white short-sleeved T-shirt with navy and white plaid shorts. The other, appearing lanky wore his black hair slicked back, a black short-sleeve T-shirt, and blue jeans.

"Long time no see!" drawled Mr. Clean. "What do you know, Slim?"

"Not a hell of a lot, Butch. I was released a week ago after doing time for stalking my girlfriend. Imagine three years! All that I did for her, buying her clothes and a car! That bitch would rat on her own mother. I should have killed her!"

"Slim, I spent 15 years in the slammer for armed robbery including time in the hole and was just released three days ago!"

Oh, no! My heart pounded while I overheard this. How much longer would we have to ride with them? What if Butch and Slim hijacked the bus? Mother's previous words of wisdom, "We will all face uncertainties," haunted me. My life streamed before me like an endless film loop—first day at school, high school graduation, college life, first day on the job. Imagining the blood-spattered bus on the 6:00 news, I wondered, "Who would notify our families?"

If hijacking occurred, how could I escape through the window? Or should I just hide under my seat? Were other passengers planning similar escape strategies?

After an hour went by, both Slim and Butch quaffed liquor from flasks hidden under their seats, then hollered," Yippee Ki-yay!" bent on annoying other passengers. Believing that they were God's gifts to women, both staggered through the aisles, slurring, "Hey, senorita, how about a little kiss?" while reeking of alcohol and body odor.

We all cowered in our seats, not knowing if those men were armed or toying with us. Suddenly the driver sped into a parking lot of the Gaylord, Michigan police post. "I know about you guys. Pipe down or the next time I'll throw you off the bus before you even get to Saginaw!"

Darn it! Three more hours with them! I repeatedly prayed the Mother of Perpetual Help novenas, and the prayers to St. Michael the Archangel and to Jude, Saint of the Impossible. All the while, several of the passengers pretended to doze. Given my thimble bladder, I even broke a record of not needing the restroom for four hours that day!

Finally, we arrived in Saginaw, Slim and Butch's destination. Former hostages, in a sense, yelling "Hallelujah," we rejoiced at being unharmed and released from our own prison. During the remainder of the trip to Kalamazoo, however, my insides still shook, and I suffered a splitting headache. What a story for Mom and Dad!

The next day, Dad complained to the bus company and the Alpena State Police Post. "I understand there were two released prisoners on the Greyhound bus from Alpena yesterday. Why were they riding unescorted?"

"Well, they did their time, so they are free."

"Since those thugs bragged so much about their former crimes, the passengers were afraid of being potential victims. My visually impaired daughter was also on that bus. If she suffered any physical harm, you'd have to incarcerate me, too, because I'd break every bone in their bodies!"

Dad took his case to city council and encouraged me, "Sandy, You're good at this. Write letters to our state senators and representatives to tell them about this incident and their need to amend the laws more in favor of protecting the public. We will fight for our rights!"

These were tough lessons regarding galvanization of emotions into constructive action. faith, relief, and gratitude in being physically unharmed, and forgiveness seared into my memory.

Again, by being a worrywart, I initially wobbled in faith which strengthened as I trusted more in God.

Faith Conquers All

"Sandy, before you leave, I need to explain several things to you," Dr. Melluish said after my annual eye examination on March 2, 1995. "You have a very thick cataract in your left eye and a rapidly developing one in your right eye. This year I should operate on your !eft eye to rule out any complications before I operate on your right eye which you depend upon for mobility and reading next year."

Taken aback, I stammered, "C-couldn't I d-delay the operation for another year? Is it really that necessary?"

"Ah! You think I'm trying to talk you into surgery! Well, it is your decision." Dr. Melluish continued. "But what if you were to lose more vision in the immediate future? Then you'd really be stuck for a while with two bad eyes."

My stomach churned and my head spun. No wonder around Christmastime, any lighting such as traffic lights, automobile headlights, and Christmas displays including candles lit during Midnight Mass seen at a distance appeared double! So, that also explained why people and objects seen through my left eye became increasingly blurry as if looking through yellow sunglasses! This caused me much difficulty in distinguishing colors; for example, pink, red, and blue to me appeared as peach, orange, and green.

Fear of dying from anesthesia intensified during a flashback of myself as a four-year-old child lying on the operating table before undergoing a tonsillectomy 42 years ago. Strangers who appeared like otherworldly aliens dressed in odd shower caps, gowns, and masks closed in on me while I fought a mask pressed tightly over my face and the sickening smell of ether before I went under.

Born with retinopathy of prematurity, I also wondered what my chances would be for a successful cataract surgery. Reading my thoughts, the doctor patted me on the shoulder and said, "Today, even in your case, with modern surgical techniques, the outcome is pretty darn good, anywhere from 95% to 97% success rate. I would not recommend surgery unless you could benefit from it."

During the next several weeks, apprehension regarding the operation clung to me like an albatross. What would I have done without the prayerful and emotional support from family, friends, and coworkers who lit candles at mass for my intentions and included me on their church prayer lists? Encouraging me, Mother said, "Jesus helped you get through school and college and find a job. He'll get you through this, too." Dad and my brother-in-law tried teasing the bugbears out of me, but like Thomas in the Bible who questioned Jesus' resurrection after death when informed of it, I remained skeptical regarding my surgical outcome.

Meditating on our Lord's Passion during Good Friday services intellectually pulled me into perspective. My sufferings would be minute compared with those of Jesus. If Jesus who so loved the world and his Father suffered a heinous death on a cross to redeem humanity, then I could certainly face this operation scheduled for May 16 at Borgess Hospital in Kalamazoo. The childhood trauma still haunted me emotionally until my preoperative conference with the doctor who answered all my questions regarding surgery and anesthesia. "Now don't get so wound up over this," Dr. Melluish simultaneously scolded and teased me. "Think how much better you'll see. But I know you! Telling you not to worry is like telling a fire not to burn."

On May 16, I entered the hospital buoyed by God watching over me, my parents' and sister's presence, prayers for a successful outcome, and Dr. Melluish's reassurance. "We'll take good care of you!" before the operation.

The next day I both eagerly and anxiously awaited my post-operative visit with Dr. Melluish. When asked to read the eye chart, to my astonishment, I could clearly see the big E and letters S and L on the second line of chart with my operated eye. What a far cry from only barely seeing the murky big E in March! Thank God!

Chairs in one of the doctor's waiting rooms were the same blue and mauve pastel colors I remembered before the onset of the cataract. Checking the lights in the reception area, I exclaimed, "No more double vision!" Imagine my elation upon having a clear view of buildings and trees through the lobby windows and seeing employees in Dr. Melluish's office again as human beings instead of blurry blobs running around. Hugging me, Mother said, "I told you you'd do fine!"

However, both euphoria and gratitude were distant memories in September, 1996, a month before scheduled cataract surgery on my right eye, formerly my better one. Crossing Howard Street in Kalamazoo while walking to work one morning, I noticed lights on Walk/Don't Walk signs appearing more blurred with that eye than they were a month ago. I could not see cars until they approached inches toward me. While I inched with pounding heart across the street, cars suddenly whizzed past me, missing me by the grace of God in retrospect. Even though I was traveling with a white cane, a motorist yelled, "Watch where you're going!" while others honked their horns. Eventually, another pedestrian helped me across.

Meanwhile, even with the assistance of hand magnifiers and Magic, a program magnifying material read on the computer screen, I had considerable difficulty filing and proofreading reports I transcribed from tape. Unable to read newsprint and the telephone directory even with the close circuit TV, I temporarily applied for Directory Assistance Exemption of Charges through the telephone company and discontinued the newspaper subscription, relying on televised local and national news broadcasts and Newsline for the Blind. It is a program through the National Federation of the Blind that allows access to newspapers and magazines, through touchtone telephones, portable players, mobile aps on iPhone, iPad, and iPod. I also received talking books and magazines through the State of Michigan Library for the Blind and Physically Handicapped.

Concerns about surgical risks resurfaced. "Oh, God!" I prayed one evening before bedtime, "How will I get through this month?"

"For I know the plans I have for you, plans to give you a future of hope." (Jeremiah 29:11)

How could something like trusting in God that seemed so simple be so difficult? Was God reassuring me everything would be all right after all?

The next day I asked Paul Glatz, Center Director, when I could see him. "I have an hour available now before staff meeting," he said. "Come in." Though he was not my immediate supervisor, I could easily confide my problems and aspirations to him.

"Paul, I'm can barely see well enough to file and proofread now. I'm concerned about backlog upon returning to work."

"Sandy, just do what you can. I'll ask my secretary, Linda Peterson, to help you with your work."

Somehow, calmness that I had never felt for most of the summer swept over me like a warm balm healing my heart. People were also praying for my speedy recovery. Following this successful cataract surgery on my right eye, how ecstatic I was to continue reading and other daily tasks before the onset of cataracts and that my visual acuity returned from 20/400 to 20/200 as it used to be! Losing vision to cataracts taught me not to take it for granted anymore.

As the Apostles on the Road to Emmaus initially did not recognize Jesus following the Resurrection. I, too, failed to recognize His Presence in the above situations. Yet, as Scripture says, He is the same today, yesterday, and tomorrow. Why was I so slow to grasp this?

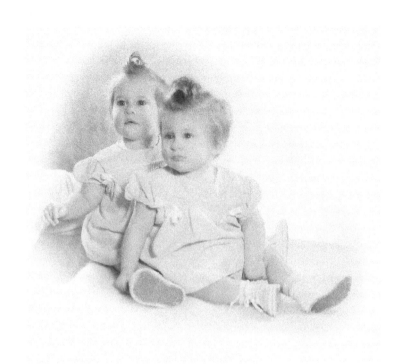

Nancy and me (front), Summer 1949.

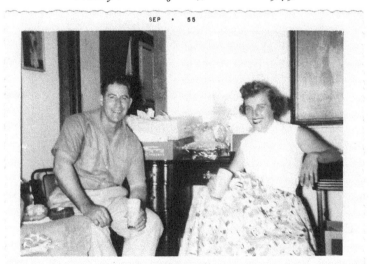

Paquette Wedding Rehearsal: Dad and Mom, August, 1955.

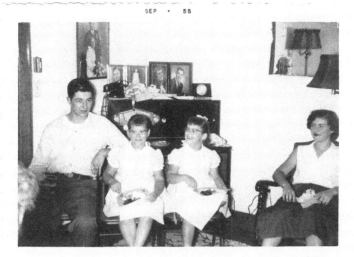

SEP · 55

Paquette Wedding Rehearsal: Nancy and me (right).

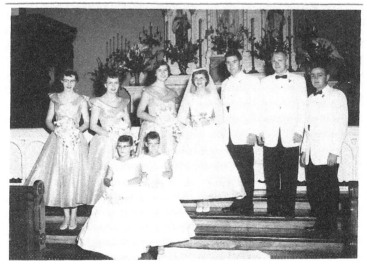

Flower Girls at the Paquette Wedding: I am on the left.

87

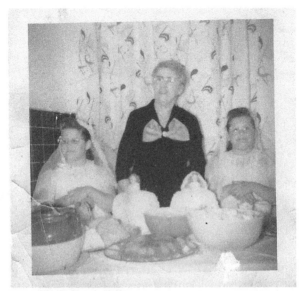

First Communion: Me (left), Grandma "Foster"/Fortier,
Nancy, May, 1957.

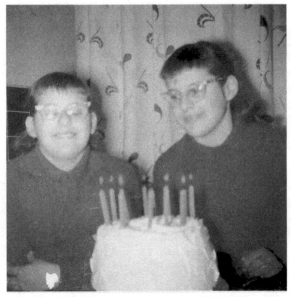

11th Birthday: I am on the right, February, 1960.

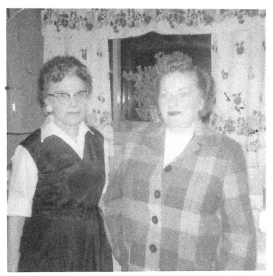

Aunt Vina (glasses) and her daughter Lillian, March, 1962.

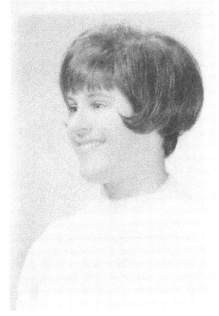

Alpena High School Graduation 1967.

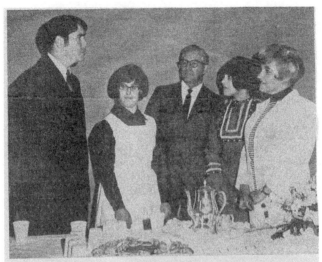

ACC COMMENCEMENT TEA — Donald Perigo, dean of student affairs at Alpena Community College greets Sandy Jo Fortier; her father, Joe Fortier; twin sister, Nancy Jo; and Mrs. Fortier. Sandy and Nancy graduated Saturday and will attend Michigan State University in September. The Fortiers reside at 123 Blair.

Alpena Community College Commencement 1969.

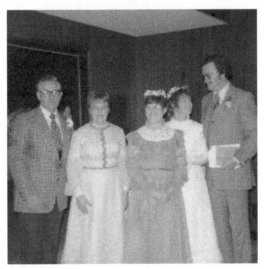

Nancy's and John's Wedding, October, 1973.

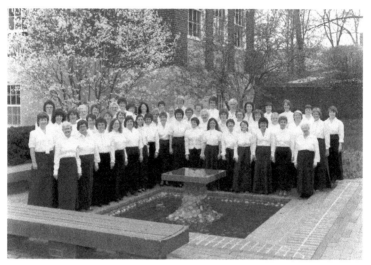

Kalamazoo Community Chorale: I am in the over blouse,
May, 1984.

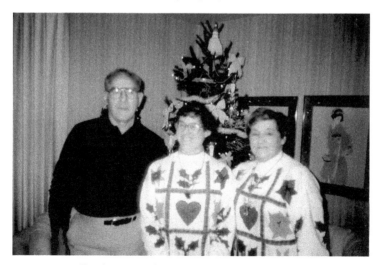

Dad, me and Mom, Christmas, 1989.

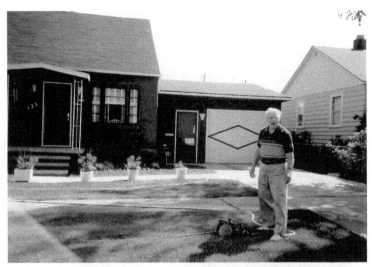

Dad is the Nicest Bloom of Summer—Alpena Home, 1995.

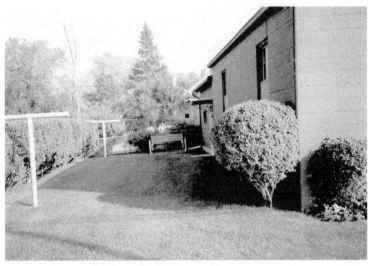

Backyard of Alpena Home, 1995.

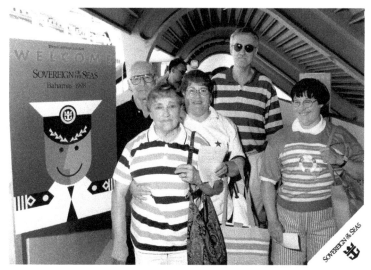

50th and 25th Fortier/Fezzey Wedding Anniversary Cruise, 1998.

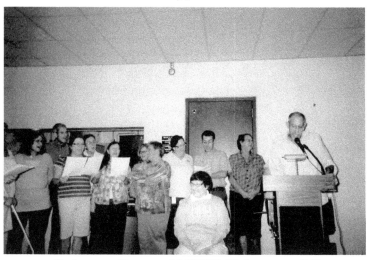

Retirement Party at MCBTC, Kalamazoo, MI, September, 2010.

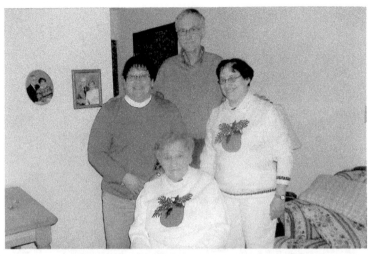

Last Photo of Mom in her Apartment, Christmas 2010.

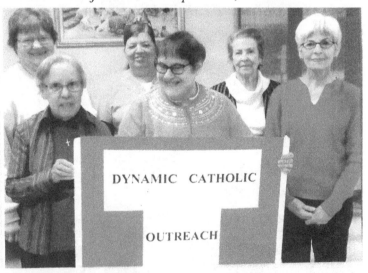

Going Away Party—Dynamic Catholic Friends—1st row left to right: Carol Raczkowski, me, Dora Kimberly—2nd row left to right: Mary Ann Redmond, Sue Rayman, Constancia Cesar, February, 2018.

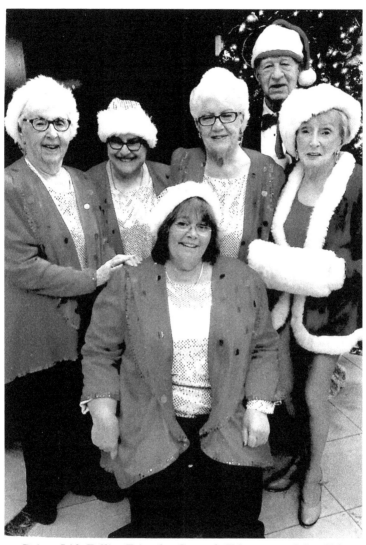

Prime Life Follies Friends, Carmel, IN—center Meredith Bovin, 1st row: Bonnie Kincaid, me, Joyce Washburn, and Lori Mansell-Solinski. "Last but not Least" Ed Solinski, December, 2018.

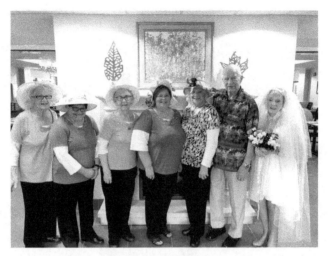

Prime Life Follies Friends—Joyce Washburn, me, Bonnie Kincaid, Meredith Bovin, Kathy Doyle, Ed Solinski and Lori Mansell-Solinski, Spring, 2019.

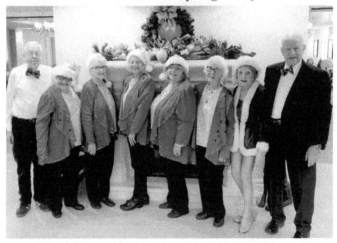

Prime Life Follies Friends, Carmel, IN, left to right—Charles Callery, me, Joyce Washburn, Kathy Doyle, Meredith Bovin, Bonnie Kincaid, Lori Mansell-Solinski and Ed Solinski, December, 2019.

CHAPTER 10: OPTIONS INTO OPPORTUNITIES

Every night before bedtime, I fervently prayed, "God, please inspire me at work. Always protect me from the hoodlums, reckless drivers, and storms. Also guide me to good, decent people." Sure enough, He orbited me from my comfort zone into experiences I had never imagined, as well as friendships that enriched my life.

Panel Discussions

For two years, in response to invitations from Western Michigan University Department of Blind Rehabilitation, Paul Glatz, Educational Director, and his wife Karen, a rehabilitation teacher at the Center, encouraged me to accompany them in speaking to prospective rehabilitation teachers about our personal and public reactions to visual impairment. In her presentation, Karen informed us that due to her poorly developed rods and cones which determined lack of color in the retina, everything appeared to her like a black-and-white movie. Noticing how Karen's classmates made fun of her coloring objects such as grass blue or purple because she could not detect the appropriate colors, Karen's teacher labeled colors in big letters on crayons. As time went on, Karen learned adaptive independent skills, including sewing Braille color tags in her clothes. Her childhood experiences had motivated her to teach blind adults. Reflecting on Karen Glatz's presentation, I often thank God for His miracle of intact color vision. How He must have wanted me to enjoy nature's splendor! This thought never struck me when I was younger.

Only being allowed several minutes to answer questions asked by each student honed a needed skill of thinking on my feet, an asset in social and work situations. Furthermore, I thank Paul Glatz for his confidence in me and Emma Evarts for encouraging me to speak as she often declared, "The ability to express oneself well both in speaking and writing is the hallmark of an intelligent person."

As well as speaking at Western Michigan University, I participated in panel discussions held at Employment Readiness seminars in March 1978, and in January, 1998, later evolving into Employment Seeking Skills and finally Employment Sales Programs. Questions for panelists listed by the coordinators or posed by the audience dealt with eye conditions, types of jobs held, duties performed, training required, challenges encountered while training and employment interviewing, and advice for individuals seeking employment. Having already described these narrated events of my panel presentations in Chapter 8, here I will only add some advice to those seeking employment:

- Pray a lot. Prayer fortified me and played a vital role in leading me to the right job and respectable co-workers.
- Explore as many vocations as you can in school and crystallize your goals, while heeding counselors' advice to explore vocational options, which I should have done, before job searching. Setting my mind on teaching as the only goal, for instance, I floundered for a while when that door slammed shut.
- Attend Employment Sales Programs which I wish were available when I was seeking employment. They would have given me valuable guidelines on job leads and appropriate questions to ask employers regarding job qualifications, advancement, wages, financial stability of businesses, their products, and services. Even employment specialists' mock interviews would have taught me how to answer tough questions more adeptly instead of answering, "Oh, anything will do," which shunted me into dead-end jobs I refused to accept.

- Sitting on an employment sales/readiness panel dais today, I would have also mentioned electronic application for state and federal civil service employment. This process would have included downloading or investigating a 12-month trial appointment application for people with disabilities if none were available in lieu of taking an exam, downloading, and saving multiple versions of the application tailored for various jobs. Online information, too, would have included job specifications, pay, résumé, cover letter and interviewing tips, scheduled examinations, and career path charts. Also investigate federal and state civil service study guides on the internet, libraries, and in bookstores for practice tests to simulate the actual one.

- Seek the services of job coaches, such as those employed by Bosma Enterprises, a blind rehabilitation and job training program in Indianapolis, Indiana. Job coaches counsel new employees, their teammates, and their manager to improve acceptance of blindness and employees' functioning abilities in the workplace. The assistance of a job coach often includes working with an employer's information technology team to obtain the necessary computer technology and orient employees to their work environment.

Though Betty Jacobs and the instructors enthusiastically supported me as a novice, I understood how their own work occupied most of their time. Therefore, in this case, I would have received more individual attention from a job coach.

Organizations for the Blind

Acting upon Betty Jacobs' suggestion to become a member of the Michigan Association for the Blind as a social outlet and means of advocating for the blind, I joined MAB in September, 1973, holding the office of secretary from January, 1974 until June, 1976. Secretarial responsibilities involved taking minutes of monthly meetings and sending announcements and news releases publicizing those meetings to local radio stations and the *Kalamazoo Gazette.*

Since the meetings were held on the first Friday of the month, I eventually became a member-at-large, reluctant to be confined on Friday meetings, because my parents frequently visited me on weekends. Had I delved as deeply as I do now into issues of blindness, I would have contributed more passionately to this organization.

I shall never forget the statewide MAB convention held in Lansing during the weekend of October 24-26, 1975, at Olds Plaza Hotel. Though I have taken the bus to visit my parents in Alpena, how excited I was at this trip to Lansing! Talking Book Radio at Michigan State University scheduled tours of the station and ten-minute taped interviews featuring conventioneers. How proud I was to have been included in that special program broadcast two weeks later! Though I would have better understood the origin of all the motions presented had I reviewed the agenda beforehand, I soon realized the importance of bylaws in convention business meetings, and I enjoyed socializing at the banquet.

Mentor Momentum

Marilyn Rubin, a former supervisor at the Michigan Commission for the Blind Training Center, exemplified the definition of a mentor as a person who supervises a less-experienced employee, shares experience and expertise to help that employee set goals and solve problems. Arriving like a needed rain shower on dry grass, she sensed that I had been stagnating in my work, only thermoforming Braille materials, transcribing from rough draft and/or tapes, and filing. Despite my willingness to assume greater responsibility, people who recognized my visual limitations doubted my abilities. However, I do not blame them, because I did not assert myself very well then, either.

While other people dismissed my further education as merely book learning, Marilyn encouraged me to continue taking courses as a launching pad to advancement into the secretarial field. To help me overcome previous difficulty with screening and transferring calls using the Centrex phone system, Marilyn devised a simple-step practice technique where she called me and requested that I transfer her calls to various locations in the building, praising lavishly but sincerely and encouraging me to be more assertive. Under her supervision, my self-confidence and enthusiasm for my work finally blossomed.

Secretarial Courses and Seminars

Goaded by the Holy Spirit's inspiration via Marilyn Ruben's mentorship and the support of family and friends that He placed in my path, the carrot of advancement, and the stick of skeptics between 1975 and 2008, I continued secretarial courses in addition to Office Machines and Office Procedures at Alpena Community College, Hadley School for the Blind Correspondence Courses, and technology in-service training at MCBTC. This included Kalamazoo Public School adult education courses in bookkeeping, business law, accounting, business math, as well as Kalamazoo Valley Community College courses in Business English, Business Principles and Practices, and Computer Usage. In the meantime, the Michigan Department of Civil Service, Professional Secretaries International, and Western Michigan University offered seminars on the role of administrative support in blind rehabilitation, telephone, and communication techniques, delivering effective presentations, problem solving, time and stress management, Word Perfect, Windows XP, and Microsoft Word. Though I found all courses stimulating, sign language proved the most challenging, since learning all the signs required spelling them in my hand. However, that course did eventually benefit me in communicating more effectively with deaf-blind students at MCBTC and in signing "Cover the World with Love," during a concert with other Kalamazoo Community Chorale members.

Professional Secretaries International

Through information obtained from Western Michigan University secretarial seminars and a neighbor's encouragement to develop more self-confidence and leadership skills, I joined the local chapter of Professional Secretaries International (or PSI) on September 10,

1984. During that magical initiation, the candle lit signi-
fied eternal glow of increased personal and professional
strengths that new members bring to the organization.
Finally, consideration as a professional bolstered my
self-esteem and interest in serving on committee projects. Before long, I submitted outlines of my own study
resources for the CPS examination in our local chapter
and Michigan Division newsletters, gathered samples of
promotional products from various office supply vendors, collated handouts, and stuffed these materials into
PSI seminar attendees' folders.

In addition, I assisted our local PSI chapter in hosting
a Michigan Division Association meeting. This involved
investigating entertainment possibilities for the Saturday
evening banquet, donating baked goods served during
conference breaks, and greeting guests at the MDAM
convention. Later, serving on the Friendship Committee, I sent sympathy and get-well cards to PSI members.

Now the organization name has changed to "International Association of Administrative Professionals".

*Volunteering and/or Participation in Center-Related Projects
and Potlucks*

Proving myself in this PSA supportive environment
launched me into volunteering for Center projects,
such as contributing household items and goodies for
our annual fund-raising charity Christmas auctions and
conducting a Thanksgiving food drive for Kalamazoo
Loaves and Fishes. I enjoyed singing at occasional talent
shows organized by the staff.

Upon staff instigation at one summer picnic since
there were not many willing volunteers, I accepted the
challenge of going through the Bounce House maze but
got caught in the bottleneck, a narrow opening toward
the end of the maze. I tried to wriggle through but to no
avail. Backing into the maze, I further engulfed myself
in the plastic. I still don't know how Betty Lujan-Roberts
pulled me out.
I was literally the butt of staff jokes because when I got
caught, my derriere reared up. I'm still chuckling now

as I recall it. That's where I earned my reputation for being rowdy at Center events!

I especially enjoyed preparing dishes to pass. Most of the fun lay in tasting different foods at summer and auction potlucks. Who could forget Renate's jelly rolls, Aggie's cheesy potato bake, or Rose's sweet potato pie? Yes, we worked hard but also had fun. No wonder I dubbed the Center staff as my second family!

CPS Certification

"How can a visually impaired person expect to pass the CPS exam under the same conditions as a normally sighted person? Impossible!" scoffed a neighbor. Despite this skepticism, I was determined to beat the odds of becoming a Certified Professional Secretary and, therefore, challenged others to do the same.

Spurred on by brochures and dynamic speakers promoting the Certified Professional Secretary designation while I attended an annual Professional Secretary Seminar at Western Michigan University in 1976, I regarded sitting for the CPS exam as another challenge to surmount like learning to read print, ride a bike, or operate a computer. As kerosene fuels fire, loving, loyal support from family, other secretaries, and CPS review course instructors at Kalamazoo Valley Community College already sparked my inherent drive to succeed in this endeavor.

From that day on, preparing for the CPS exam involved ten years of diligent studying with a close circuit TV magnifier. As well as college courses previously mentioned, I perused Plaid and Wiley Series Workbooks and available recommended recorded books from the State of Michigan Library for the Blind and Physically Handicapped. I also attended civil service seminars related to CPS exam topics.

A co-worker remarked, "If God wills, you will pass." Navigating me through school, college, and employment, He also called on people as His instruments to assist me in applying for CPS certification, namely then the Center director, Paul Glatz. Initially, he reacted with a mixture of pride and reservation.

As time went by, Paul's growing concerns regarding my CPS qualifications and possible rejection subsequently led him to contact PSI Headquarters for more information. Apparently, according to my civil service classification, my work experience did not coincide with the PSI Headquarters' specifications of a secretary working for one boss and performing an array of duties requiring considerable judgment. After a two-hour telephone consultation, Paul informed me that my courses taken would qualify me for the required secretarial experience. Praise God for a caring intervener to PSI Headquarters and for their acceptance!

He did not stop there. Throughout the exam, God also planted another human angel over my shoulder, a proctor with the gentle demeanor of a nun who quelled test jitters by reassuring and praying for all examinees. Consequently, peace enveloped me during this test. To my surprise, unanticipated answers to tough questions also emerged. Again, I thank God for directing me to excellent instructors who prepared me for this exam. In 1983, I passed Behavioral Science in Business, Economics and Management, and Office Technology on the first attempt. In 1985, I passed Accounting/Business Law and Business Communications, and in 1986, Office Administration, completing the CPS Exam.

As the organization of Professional Secretaries International evolved into International Association of Administrative Professionals, the former CPS exam I had taken is now renamed Certified Administrative Professional (CAP) Exam. Candidates for the CAP exam must apply online for eligibility and accommodations. For further information, type International Association of Administrative Professionals or IAAP as search engines.

Call for Papers and Other Submissions

God, the Holy Spirit often motivates us indirectly through the people we meet and directly through our sensations and emotions. This was apparent one day when He nudged me to write, beginning with a submission to "Call for Papers" coordinating with The Secretary Speakout. Hesitation and Bible admonitions about the man who buried his talent in the ground increased my emotional tension.

This strange feeling vanished after I submitted the paper, "Self-Image and the Professional Secretary." To my surprise, the required abstract of the paper I had also written appeared in the March, 1985, edition of *The Secretary*:

"Progress has been made by many secretaries and their supervisors in upgrading the image of the professional secretary, yet unfavorable attitudes toward the profession still exist—because of the social conditioning of women to think of themselves and their work as second class and the lack of integrity among secretaries themselves. Survival basically depends upon an unswerving belief in contributions to work and society."

Amplifying these abstract themes throughout the paper, my unpublished personal experiences exemplified the nurturing roles family, supervisors, and coworkers played to build high self-esteem. I included how I dispelled unfavorable public perceptions of me as a secretary by performing my best, upholding my own moral principles, taking courses, and deflecting negative comments with positive ones toward the profession.

In the 1987 Secretary Speakout, my paper, "Technology: Creating and Fulfilling Dreams of Aspiring Visually Impaired Secretaries," lauded the development of modern technology and low-vision devices for its impact in opening doors for the blind and partially seeing like me into secretarial employment.

Again, God impelled me to respond to the 1993 Secretary Call for Papers and Speakout. Regarding the topic, "The 21st Century Secretary," I submitted my story about attaining the CPS and motivating other blind and visually impaired people to do the same.

Michigan Commission for the Blind Newsletter, The Tilt

Buoyed by these previous Professional Secretaries International publications and swept up in the fervor and pride shared with other Michigan Commission for the Blind staff who created a newsletter called *The Tilt*, I submitted the poem entitled "Visually Impaired" illustrated below:

Visually Impaired

The other day I got done swimming at the Y,
I met a mother inwardly beautiful, smart, and
Filled with a loving heart.
Her little boy asked, "Why does that lady walk with
   a white cane?
Is she in pain?"
The mother replied, "Perhaps she is,
Because she cannot see.
I don't know how that came to be.
But I do know, Tommy,
That God made us all special,
Including those of us who can't walk, talk,
Hear, think, or see."
What is it like to be blind or partially sighted?
This is a subject on which I must dwell.
Sometimes it is hard to tell what it is like
Just by looking at people.
Living with blindness or limited vision,
Either congenital or adventitious,
Can be much like meandering
Through a crazy funhouse consisting
Of dark rooms filled with cobwebs of gloom,
And drop-offs, and whirligigs, and chutes tripping
   people up,
And mirrors reflecting
Some images that seem larger,
Others smaller,
Some taller,
Others shorter,
Some fatter,
Others skinnier
Than what the average person sees.
Facing the future as a newly visually impaired
   person, I pondered
And often wondered,
"How will our world so shattered
Have ever mattered
To the normal crowd?"
Trying to describe it to them
Is like explaining why
Everything is dark,

Colors are more faded,
The ocean is deeper,
Steps are much steeper
Halls appear narrower or wider
Or other things seem nearer or farther to us
Than they do to the rest of the world.
Having no vision or partial sight
Is a feeling of
Being locked into a closet or box
Enveloped by darkness or dim light
From floor to ceiling.
Sometimes poor vision resembles
A pair of shackles
Bound ever so tight,
Even challenging Houdini's might!
Am I raising anyone's hackles
By implying that I'm giving up the fight?
Heavens, no!
Like a baseball player just up to bat
I shall not give up just like that!
I, Hanna Huggles,
Did hope and can finally cope with life's struggles
   and rigor,
Filled with the recently acquired vigor,
Thanks to Center staff
Which have crossed my path!
With so much firmness yet kindness,
They have shown me that
One does live a fulfilling life
Despite blindness!
As a happy ending to my story,
Now I can glory
Turning past tragedy into triumph!

Americans with Disabilities Act (ADA) Essay Contest and Campaign

Where would we be without the Americans with Disabilities Act? Accolades to all legislators who voted and to President Bush who signed this into law on July 26, 1990! How elated and proud Louis Braille, Anne Sullivan, and Helen Keller would have been if they lived to see ADA enacted in their lifetimes!

How could I show my appreciation to these legislators and to President Bush? Ten years later, an answer struck me again with the Holy Spirit's prompting through flyers circulating around MCBTC which advertised an essay contest on the topic of the Americans with Disabilities Act (ADA) sponsored by the National Organization on Disabilities and Senator Harkin's Campaign, "Day in the Life of ADA." As one of countless participants, I zealously submitted the following essay with a cover letter introducing myself and summarizing my difficulties with seeking employment already detailed in Chapter 8.

ADA: America's Gain

"America! Land of Opportunity!" President Bush's signing into law the Americans with Disabilities Act ten years ago has perpetuated our cherished legacy by giving disabled persons the chance to do things most other people normally take for granted, such as grocery shopping, purchasing clothes in the malls, eating out, attending concerts, plays, and museums, and banking. Thanks to barrier-free public buildings containing wide aisles, wheelchair-accessible bathrooms, and elevators, or ramps, and, in many cities, Dial-A-Ride vans equipped with wheelchair lifts. Museums offer large-print handouts, Braille tour guides, taped descriptions of exhibits, tactile exhibits, and telecommunications devices for the deaf. Many banks have provided large-print checks and registers, and some are also installing talking ATMs for the blind and dyslexic. Braille and large-print menus and Braille numbers on elevators have allowed blind and visually impaired people to choose their own meals and ascend and descend elevators more independently.

ADA has launched new employment opportunities as exemplified by developmentally disabled baggers at grocery stores and retail establishments. Former multiply disabled consumers of the Michigan Commission for the Blind Training Center and others like them portrayed in the news sought employment in business enterprise, teaching, law, computer programming and troubleshooting, counseling, and secretarial careers. Awareness of disabilities through ADA has given enterprising vendors, such as LS&S, Inc. and HARC Mercantile, Ltd., an ever-demanding, productive market for the myriad adaptive computers and daily living devices. Thus, accommodation and increasing employment opportunities for more disabled consumers have spurred the U.S. economy."

Imagine my delight in receiving Senator Harkin's warm, welcome, and winning acknowledgement:

"August 10, 2000

Dear Sandra:

> *Thank you for sending me your ADA story. It is hard to believe that ten years have passed since the signing of the Americans with Disabilities Act. By eliminating barriers everywhere from education to health care, from streets to public transportation, from parks to shopping malls, and from courthouses to Congress, the ADA has opened new worlds to people with disabilities. People with disabilities are participating more in their communities and living fuller lives as students, coworkers, taxpayers, consumers, voters, and neighbors.*

> *The response to my "Day in the Life of the ADA" campaign has been very encouraging and has helped me to understand what we still must do to give all Americans an equal opportunity to live out their dreams of independence. I greatly appreciate your contribution to this campaign. Please be assured that I will continue to fight for the principle that disability no way diminishes a person's right to participate in the cultural, economic, educational, political, and social mainstream.*

> *Again, thank you for sharing your views with me. Please don't hesitate to let me know how you feel on any issue that concerns you.*

> *Sincerely,*
> *Tom*
> *United States STH/mae"*

Discovery Learning

Having completed the one-day, new employee immersion training years ago, the entire Michigan Commission for the Blind Training Staff were required to complete a more extensive updated Discovery Learning course offered by Douglas C. Boone from fall of 2001 until summer of 2002. Our group underwent this tvoluntraining from June 3-7, 2002.

Simulating training at the Michigan Commission for the Blind Training Center, the first day began at the Country Inn and Suites where my blindfolded group ascended and descended stairs, found restrooms and convention rooms where Doug emphasized a problem-solving approach using distance and environmental cues such as sound, wind, the sun's heat, smell, and texture. To locate items in the restroom such as the toilet, sink, paper holder, mirror, and door, we explored our surroundings by tapping our canes and moving our hands over the walls and items. Sounds of running water or flushing toilet hinted where our positions in the room were in proximity to sink and toilet. We used similar methods of discovery training to explore a convention room, such as arcing our canes between rows of chairs and counting rows from the door leading to the back of the room. I finally realized how listening for cues and sliding the cane from side to side and up and down on stairs enables a blind person to move more confidently even without holding onto the handrails. Exhausted at day's end, I certainly did identify with students overwhelmed by training when they first arrive at the Center.

On the second day we moved on to Kalamazoo Valley Community College where we learned to identify certain classrooms while we traveled and reversed routes. Using a pencil grip on our canes enabled us to walk behind people and to locate chairs more gracefully as a mobility technique used by blind people while they attend meetings or are seated in a restaurant.

Spending several hours in residential travel and at Milham Park both with and without the occluder (or blindfold) and lunching at a Chinese restaurant on the third day, our group also learned to break the unsafe habit of only moving the cane in a straight line while traveling. Widely arcing the cane from side to side to function better in navigating sidewalks is like turning on headlights when driving to anticipate unexpected movements of people or animals. Failing to arc my cane, I would have fallen into an undetected gaping hole in the sidewalk if Doug had not caught me. Under the occluder, I also discovered that judging distance of the car motor running allows ample time to pass the driveway before the driver backs out.

On the fourth day, we crossed a busy intersection with a traffic light and devoted class time to discussing what we learned about ourselves during this training.

Graduation day consisted of ordering lunch at Wendy's: entering, ordering, obtaining, and carrying a tray full of food, and eating under occluder. Miraculously, I found a table and ate without food landing on my chest. What I learned in that week amazed me.

World Service Center and Clinton Museum and Library

Before passage of the Americans with Disabilities Act into law, rehabilitation counselors and teachers had referred students who had completed personal adjustment at the Michigan Commission for the Blind Training Center for vocational training to the World Service for the Blind (WSB), formerly known as the Lions World Service Center, in Little Rock, Arkansas, since students were guaranteed training with necessary accommodations there. During a family vacation down South in May, 2005, I finally discovered how the MCBTC and WSB programs compared while touring the World Services for the Blind, founded by Roy Kump in 1947 to teach blind and partially sighted people how to function independently in our sighted society. As I recall, WSB offered a complete personal adjustment program, nine vocational courses, a vision rehabilitation clinic and training, an assistive technology learning center, job placement assistance, and a college preparatory program. WSB is accredited by the National Accreditation Council for agencies serving people with blindness or visual impairments.

Whereas MCBTC emphasized personal adjustment training, WSB focused primarily on vocational training with teaching independent living skills as secondary. Before vocational training, students underwent a 30-day evaluation in techniques of daily living including cooking, orientation and mobility, personal grooming, home management, math, written and oral communication, personal signature, and ability to relate to people, such as supervisors, coworkers, and the public in the workplace.

WSB dorms were located upstairs and classes were on the bottom of the building whereas some dorms at MCBTC were located downstairs as well as upstairs. Otherwise WSB classrooms resembled those of MCBTC. Touring WSB finally satisfied my curiosity regarding this facility.

I also enjoyed the President William Jefferson Clinton Museum and Library. Even though the items were encased in glass, the showcase presentation allowed me to see everything up close including his speeches, his and First Lady Hillary Clinton's schedules, family photographs, elegant dinner menus, a mannequin of an evening gown Hillary wore, and pictures chronicling his presidency. Imagine even walking up to a replica of President Clinton's Oval Office! The huge Chihuly blown glass exhibit centrally located in the room which appeared like a tree consisting of twisted branches made of noodles intrigued me as the most extraordinary artwork. The Clinton Museum and Library also contains wide aisles and many audio-visual aids as other factors complying with the American Disabilities Act.

Like a fledgling robin learning to fly, I needed to spread my wings initially in a supportive, less risky atmosphere away from work. Serving on those Professional Secretaries International committees allowed me to survey and attempt various projects, gaining experience to handle similar future projects at my supervisor's request. Here, I also learned how to interact with different personalities. Oh, how the domineering ones certainly tried my patience and diplomacy!

During panel discussions, I began sharing my story about living blind in a sighted world even then. I realized how other blind people like me coped with life's challenges in various ways.

Taking secretarial/office administration courses and attaining certification as a professional secretary/administrative professional demonstrated my commitment to employee development and dispelled supervisors' doubts regarding my abilities. As a result, I later assumed greater responsibilities.

PSI Secretary Speakout Call for Papers afforded me the opportunity to express my views on specific issues affecting secretaries. It fulfilled my need to advocate for other secretaries and myself as professionals.

For the first time, I experienced the excitement of having articles published in *The Secretary* and in *The Tilt*. During this time, however, I had never seriously considered writing as a hobby or a vocation.

The ADA essay contest launched me into championing rights for people with disabilities and paying a debt of gratitude to President Bush for signing this bill into law. Again, using my experiences as illustrations, I impressed upon people how restricted their lives would have been without passage of ADA.

Through adaptive in-service staff orientation and mobility/discovery learning, I learned how to ascend and descend curbs and steps more efficiently using my cane to glide over them. I also rely more on hearing to judge the distance of car motors while crossing streets and driveways. I never forgot how touch establishes the layout of a room while I wore sleep shades.

Volunteering to conduct the Center food drive for Kalamazoo Loaves and Fishes, I gained skills in organizing the drive and delegating tasks to Center staff and students.

I also enjoyed socializing with staff at picnics. The Bounce House incident taught me to laugh at myself and take life less seriously.

Visiting the World Service Center for the Blind satisfied my curiosity regarding its services. Observing its different training approach from that of MCBTC, I have seen how WSB has led blind people into lucrative careers and independent lives.

Visiting the Clinton Museum introduced me to a vital piece of American history including hands-on views of the Oval Office, thanks to the Americans with Disabilities Act.

These opportunities expanded my horizons and enabled me to grow professionally.

CHAPTER 11: MYTHS, MILLERS, AND MOSQUITOES

Myths. How do we handle these pesky critters? Well, dodge them, accept them, or overcome them! This chapter will illustrate how my personal experience has debunked many common myths.

Heeding Dr. Ruedemann's wise advice and our own common sense, my family and I also refused to allow any myths to stereotype me as a blind person warehoused in any institution or as a spectator. Ignoring several naysayers' warnings, "Sandy will never wear glasses. She'll just yank them off," Dr. Rudemann affirmed, "I would have put glasses on her when she was six months old." To distract me from pulling off the glasses, Mother put them on me while I was drinking my favorite orange pop. In fact, I cannot remember ever being without glasses.

Knowing how I sat comfortably close to television or movie screens to clarify what I was seeing, my parents ignored relatives' admonitions of how "sitting too close to the TV will ruin her eyes."

"Feed her carrots; they're good for the eyes," others exhorted. Dr. Ruedemann scoffed, "You could feed her carrots until they give her a gut ache, but they will not increase her vision to 20/20!"

This has always amused me: "You must have been an easy child to raise. Being visually impaired, you sat all the time and didn't get into things." Quite the opposite! Limited vision increased my nosiness, taxing the patience of many adults. In fact, my parents even tried to quell it by reading me "The Elephant's Child" by Rudyard Kipling.

Wondering why film appeared like thin ribbon in its spool but so magnified in its images on the screen, I

115

wished teachers kept old films and projectors around to examine or explained in simple terms the creation of film or operation of projectors. Naturally inquisitive, I also peered into holes of iron gratings to investigate why sewers were dark and infinite.

Baffled, Mother inquired about the reasons for this behavior to Dr. Ruedemann during an appointment. "Doctor, could you please explain to me why Sandy goes so close to things? Being out in public, I'm so embarrassed when she runs up to strangers to see or feel what they are wearing."

"That's the way she learns and explores the world around her," he replied. "Moving up to objects that you and I can see at a distance or holding them up close brings them into focus for her. I'd be more concerned if she just sat passively in a chair."

I always liked exploring old buildings. Like an archeologist studying ancient Minoan/Cretan civilizations, what would I discover by tearing back layers of old wallpaper in abandoned houses? What were the families like who lived there? Why did they choose this ugly black and white plaid kitchen wallpaper? Why was that living room painted maroon with white enamel baseboards and moldings? Did the families move because the house was haunted?

Given my inquisitiveness and daring do, I persuaded Nancy to join me in exploring Christiansen's dark, mysterious antique shop. How I wanted to see and touch everything in there no matter what! Running inside, I discovered a mahogany highboy with serrated edges in a crimson room.

Then I scurried into another room. Phew! A box of encyclopedias smelling as if they had been stored in someone's damp basement for years, a cinnamon-scented candle, a pink milk glass cake plate, and tattered maps of Europe lay on one table.

A silky sampler with felt embroidered letters, "Home is Where the Heart Is," and a music box playing "Braham's Lullaby" placed on another table captured my interest. Hanging from the ceiling by the window, a chandelier with dangling prisms reflecting rainbow colors bouncing on the walls from the sun fascinated me as well. Meanwhile, Nancy was examining several old-fashioned wooden puzzles.

Suddenly a voice loomed as if from a tomb, "No children allowed!" Formerly hidden in the dusty darkness, Mr. Christianson's wizened body scuttled toward us like a brown recluse spider exposed to sunlight.

"Let's get out of here!" Nancy shoved me out of the building.

I am so happy that my parents ignored pessimists and encouraged me to take physical education in school, including swimming and bowling. In bowling, they suggested using the ball return as a frame of reference to judge not to go too near the foul line as the bowling alley employees then did not consider rails as accommodation.

Dad even installed a basketball hoop with netting and backboard on one side of the laundry lines in our backyard. Nancy and I played softball at our camp and on a summer team. This in turn helped me to develop mobility skills that I needed to gain self-confidence which I would not have had otherwise if I constantly worried about bumping into people and objects.

I've seen videos of MCBTC students at the Kalamazoo Airport who have gone skydiving in tandem with experienced skydivers. I did not aspire to those heights!

Childhood cruelty can stem from little understanding or empathy regarding limited vision as a disability. Often children enjoyed making fun of me, thinking that would not bother me because I was too stupid. What possessed Stewart, one of the neighborhood boys, to break my glasses? I'll always wonder. Perhaps he thought, "Sandy doesn't see well anyway, so glasses don't help her at all."

One day, Nancy and I were playing outside when my glasses fell. Stewart grabbed them and gleefully bent the frame so that they were no longer useful. He also broke Nancy's glasses, hitting them with snowballs. He and two other neighborhood boys loved to throw snowballs.

Hearing their Tarzan yell even before the boys entered our yard, Nancy and I should have sensed imminent trouble. I also worried about their pegging snowballs accidentally in my eyes because of potential damage. Nancy and I screamed in anger and fright.

Hearing our screams and seeing the broken glasses, Mother called Stewart's parents. To teach him a lesson, they brought with them his piggy bank to purchase new glasses. That hurt Nancy and me more than his misdeed. In fact, I cried, realizing that Stewart would be deprived of his piggy bank. Mother and Dad pleaded, "Oh, no! Give it back to Stewart! We don't need that to buy new glasses!"

Based on my immersion training at the Michigan Commission for the Blind Training Center, I can vouch that sensitivity training with the Zimmerman Low Vision Simulation Kit, if available during the 1950s, would have been a more constructive disciplinary approach than depriving Stewart of his piggy bank. The kit contains goggles simulating different types of visual impairments, pathologies, and visual field limitations. As it did for me, wearing those goggles for a week while he played and completed household chores would have impressed upon Stewart the impact of visual impairment upon daily living.

However, cruelty and crassness are more deplorable in adults who should know better. During my childhood, several out-of-town visiting relatives knowing that I didn't see well, yet quizzing, "Remember me?" or "Guess who this is!" without identifying ,themselves, remarked that I was stupid, because I did not recognize them. This really embarrassed me! Mother snapped, "No! She is not stupid, but this childish game of yours makes her feel dumb. Please stop it!" After they left, Mother consoled me, "They're the dumb ones, not you. At least they should have had enough courtesy to identify themselves. Being unable to recognize people because of your limited vision has nothing to do with intelligence."

I also bristled when strangers said, "We think you see better than you do. You're just faking blindness or using it to get attention."

These above incidents impelled me to ask Dr. Ruedemann, "Why can I read print up close and distinguish colors but can't recognize faces?"

He explained, "Sandy, fortunately and miraculously, the cones in your retina that determine color weren't affected. Without central vision, you can see the body clearly as far as the chest but faces will always be blurry. I only know of another child, a boy in Saginaw, Michigan, who can read print. Most people with retinopathy at prematurity that you have do not." To my disappointment, however, he did not tell me how to shake my negative image in the eyes of those crass relatives. Eventually, I figured how to beat them at their own game—with humor. "Whoops! Blame it on my bad eyes!"

The first time I took a bus trip organized by Western Michigan University to Stratford, Ontario, to see Gilbert and Sullivan's *The Gondoliers,* Shakespeare's *A Midsummer Night's Dream,* and *As You Like It* in 1983, the B&B owner shuddered when I left my room. "You can't travel by yourself! I'll go with you." She calmed down after I explained to her about my limited vision. I also demonstrated how a white cane helps me navigate curbs and stairs. I informed her that it identifies me as a blind person so motorists know when to stop, and how I can detect landmarks even with my limited vision. I added, "Besides, I get around in Kalamazoo, Michigan, which is bigger than Stratford. I even walk to work and take buses and cabs by myself to run errands and attend concerts." As blind persons, we must educate the public.

The assumption that a blind person is also deaf and needs an interpreter both puzzles and annoys me. For example, one of Nancy's neighbors who popped over one Christmas approached me literally in my face, waving and bellowing, "Do you see me?" I think she got the message when I backed away from her!

I could not understand why deli or restaurant servers asked my family instead of me to tell them what I wanted to order. Nancy explained that the servers could not hear me, since I mumbled while holding the menu so close to my mouth or while putting my head down as I tried to see available items in the glass deli case. Speaking more assertively and researching online menus so I can decide what to order ahead of time resolved these issues. As another solution, Nancy identifies items in the deli case for me.

Occasionally, individuals have expressed surprise at my intellectual contributions in education classes. Could it be they equate limited vision to limited brain power?

The other day, a neighbor asked me, "If you are legally blind, why don't you live in the dark?"

I explained that I have 20/200 visual acuity and the meaning of that. I do not know exactly what percentage of blind people live in darkness. I do know that fellow students in my medical transcription class at MSB and those at MCBTC could see at 20/200, light, shadows, colors, and forms. Some had tunnel vision, seeing objects as if through a tube. Many may have had enough vision to use magnifiers but were diagnosed with a visual field limitation.

People have also thought that I have a sixth sense. No, I'm not Wonder Woman endowed with extraordinary powers! I have simply learned to do tasks a different way and to rely more on my other senses and my memory.

Contrary to wide-spread belief, adjustment to blindness does not always follow a straight course as outlined below:

Initial shock and denial

Withdrawal from social activities

Sadness, anger, and self-pity

Planning coping strategies such as bowling instead of playing baseball, joining support groups or blindness organizations such as the National Federation of the Blind, enrolling in training centers for the blind to learn adaptive skills and self-acceptance as blind persons.

I agree with the analogy that grieving loss of sight is like grieving the loss of a loved one who died, having ridden this emotional roller coaster when facing vision loss to cataracts.

Self-esteem and acceptance of visual impairment flit from positive to negative as the birds in an aviary fly from perch to perch. As I recall entertaining an aunt, her daughter, and son-in-law during the summer of 1978, self-esteem inflated with pride when they commented upon a delicious meal consisting of chicken casserole, fruit salad, and Magic Bars, but it suddenly deflated when my aunt remarked, "Wow! It's something that you can live alone and can manage by yourself. You can even pour a glass of pop yourself!"

Students' MCBTC case notes I transcribed frequently documented similar fluctuation in self-esteem when a student's self-confidence soared higher than a rocket after he had received a stellar staffing report but plunged the next day after a frustrating independent study mobility lesson. Experiencing this same emotional fluctuation, another student who eagerly attempted a new pumpkin roll recipe to surprise her family expressed disappointment when the recipe flopped.

In a humorous vein, limited vision can tally pluses and minuses. Though I envied others who could sightread music, I often laughed while quipping to other church choir or Kalamazoo Community Chorale members who wonder how I can sing without seeing the director, "Being visually impaired is a blessing, because I don't see the director's grimaces when we neglect to follow dynamics in performances." Though I sometimes yearn for perfect vision, now I do not resent the challenges of visual impairment, because they have developed character. If I did not have limited vision, I could have faced something much worse.

Many people have remarked to me, "Beauty is in the eye of the beholder. If you cannot see beauty, how can you appreciate it?" To refute, God gave us four other senses: hearing, taste, smell, touch as well as sight to explore the world through different media. This idea inspired creation of the Five Senses Garden located at the Phoenix School across the field from the Center. As I remember it, the garden exuded the springtime fragrance of lilacs and hydrangeas beckoning me inside its entry curtained in summer green ivy, later transformed into autumn russet, orange, and gold, hanging on one brick wall. Robins chirped, redwing blackbirds pick-t-aleed, blue jays screeched, and crows cawed in a resounding chorus. Velvety lambs' ears and bushes in varying green shades and textures lined one wall. Like a railroad track, a chain of stones ran through the bushes and Serbian spruce.

Plants surrounded a mosaic floor with a sundial in the center. On the left of the floor, a grist mill clanged with rotating pails filling themselves with water and perpetuating the motion by turning each other upside down. An adjoining "room" contained flats of daisies, delicate lacy purplish-blue flowers, and red, white, and blue flower flats. Pink and purple impatiens wove a patchwork quilt beside the red, blue, and white flat.

Industrious but inhospitable bees buzzed while flitting from one flower to the next during pollination. Cabbage and monarch butterflies danced among the flowers.

Tomatoes, strawberries. and eggplants awaited harvesting for dinner. Someone also planted oregano, chamomile, dill, marjoram, sage, and garlic emitting mouth-watering aromas. As farmers rotate crops, gardeners alternate different plants every spring.

Like the Five Senses Garden, the lovely nature trail adjoining the bike track behind the Center wove its own enchantment for me while I walked during breaks and lunch hours. Wooden chips marked the trail with a fragrance of cedar and the spongy texture of carpet. How I loved that cedar aroma and wished to store it in a bottle to be released to my heart's desire at home! A hollowed-out log doubled as a comfortable table setting for me as I savored a tasty picnic lunch while absorbing all sights, sounds, fragrances, and textures of this nature trail on a summer day. Oh, to spend all day there instead of working!

Beauty does not primarily exist in my eyes but lies within my imagination and associations. To me, musical compositions performed in concert elicit a whole gamut of emotions, tastes, smells, movements, and textures. For instance, Scott Joplin's ragtime pieces evoke memories of a musty, upright, honky-tonk piano consisting of uncovered hammers and strings which captured my interest as a ten-year-old. Bluegrass music stimulates recollections of pungent hay smell and laughter on a hayride. Woodwind and brass quintets warm my heart like a heavy woolen sweater warms the body on a winter day. Organ pieces in different tonal registers roar like a bonfire or erupt like volcanoes spewing molten lava. A piano piece refreshes me like a cold glass of sugar-free lemonade. A piece for the string section in a symphony orchestra chiseled in legato, staccato, and pizzicato movements may suggest to me smooth, serrated, and slivered frosty-glass textures of an intricate ice sculpture at a winter carnival.

A little whimsy inspired me to compose this essay.

Nature's Music

During summer days and nights, trilling of birds and buzzing of insects treat me to concerts as beautiful, if not more so, than outdoor ones performed by the Indianapolis Symphony Orchestra. On summer evenings, sounds of various insects, including crickets, and katydids, outside my window lull me to sleep.

On summer mornings, I enjoy hearing the clear, piccolo-like songs of the many birds ushering in a new day. Summertime's early mornings also fill me with serenity aroused by the music of the cool, morning wind rustling through the trees at sunrise and the distant barking of a dog heralding the new day of promise. Summer mornings and evenings offer me unique sounds of nature which attune me to the awesomeness of my Father's world, uplifting my spirit, yet also providing me a haven of peace.

Thanking God for hearing and sound, which compensate for what I don't see also applies to one Fourth of July when the neighbors geared up for their grand firework finale which ended up as ear-shattering explosions without any spectacular colors. I joked, "Fireworks aren't for sighted only. Even the visually impaired can enjoy their banging, crackling, and whistling." Mother teased, "You're nuts! But I never thought of that in this way, either."

Contrary to popular opinion, I enjoy movies. Seeing *West Side Story*, for instance, I can hear the rivals between the gangs by dissonance and syncopation of Leonard Bernstein's background music. The same applies to other movies with background music. Measures of "In the Mood" may hint that the story occurs in the 1940s as another example. Someone narrates the action for me, or I research theaters online which have a special program providing audio description of the film. Heard through headphones, the audio description does not distract other patrons. When I attend plays, I reserve a seat close to the stage.

Reflecting upon other people's, as well as my own reaction to misconceptions about blindness and eager to share my experiences and insights with the young people attending a 2008 summer program at the Michigan Commission for the Blind Training Center, I conducted a one-hour seminar for them entitled, "Myths, Millers, and Mosquitoes." Launching it, I inquired, "What myths about blindness bother you? As we use Off or electronic Bug Zappers to repel and kill millers and mosquitoes on summer nights, what myth repellent do you use?"

We had a lively discussion about sighted persons' perplexity regarding why a low-vision person can see certain items clearly but not others. Adding to the discussion, I explained why I could read print but could not recognize people. I also relayed an incident of traveling downtown without a white cane on one occasion and asking a bus driver to help me locate the Westnedge Avenue bus home. He shouted, "Hey, stupid, can't you read?" Not allowing him to get away with rudeness, I reported him to the bus company.

Some students mentioned that people telling them they were stupid, clumsy, unattractive, or unable to get a job irritated them. Others attending regular classes said they felt sad and self-conscious when classmates teased them for poor physical agility, wearing heavy glasses, and using other low-vision devices, such as a monocular.

Others reacting to similar circumstances suggested analyzing how true people's comments were, taking them with a grain of salt, or throwing them over the shoulder.

One feisty student described how a bus driver stopped a block out of her destination and an elderly man then pestered her, asking her if she needed help. Wary of him and annoyed by his behavior, she exclaimed, "I can get there myself! I'll show you!" to his and other onlookers' astonishment.

Another student attending regular high school classes illustrated how assertiveness as her myth repellent gained respect from her formerly condescending teacher who decided to exempt her from taking a midterm exam after she spent many hours studying for it. I faced a similar situation with a psychology instructor at Alpena Community College. Both of us demanded the chance to prove ourselves. After all, we asserted, if we continued in higher education or transitioned into employment, our professors or supervisors would expect us to fulfill our responsibilities.

Envious classmates jeered, "You're crazy!" Perhaps we were, but we chose to champion our integrity in fulfilling our course requirements.

In the remaining time, I asked students, "Why do we internalize myths that the sighted public imposes upon us?" Someone joked, "Some of us are gullible, believing everything people tell us."

"You're right!" I affirmed. "Considering our seminar theme, that reminds me of walking into a mosquito-infested area without repellent or like allowing our mosquito bites to itch without applying any ointment for relief. Any other ideas about internalizing myths?"

Someone else stated, "Some people's mental laziness or just plain indifference regarding any issues affecting their life."

"That's true," I stated. "Some people react to life like zombies. It's so sad!"

Looking at my watch, I sighed, "I wish we had more time to pursue this topic on internalizing myths as a group. Since we don't, I suggest you continue to think about it and discuss it among yourselves. When we combat these myths, we maintain our personal dignity. This requires educating and asserting ourselves with the sighted public."

When I recapped, "In summary, what do myths, millers, and mosquitoes have in common?" the students quipped, "They bite!" "Indeed, they do," I replied, "but instead of letting myths bother us, we can empower ourselves by debunking them and moving forward to accomplish great things in our lives." I shall never forget those students' enlightening humor and insight packed into this seminar.

CHAPTER 12: THE RECKONING

Growing up accustomed to stories with happy endings, I often envisioned how these stories would represent life. For example, I imagined my aging parents enjoying the same robust health as they did when they were young or living forever. But what unsuspecting curveballs life threw, shattering this illusion!

For me, August 9, 2002, began as an ordinary day at work Brailling student schedules for the following week until the telephone rang with my sister's choking voice at the other end of the line, "I don't know how to break this more gently. Dad is in Borgess Hospital with a stroke. He and Mother were returning from errands and just pulling into their carport when he spoke of feeling funny and not being able to see. Mother called the ambulance and had him admitted into Borgess Hospital." Assured that Nancy and John were on their way and alerting my supervisor as to what occurred, I immediately returned home.

Shocked and disturbed seeing Dad in bed, I never believed he would ever walk again or that Mother and I could take care of him at home since he needed two burly aides to lift him. Fortunately, according to the speech therapist and several other doctors, he tested as a candidate for an acute physical therapy program in a wing at Borgess Hospital and follow-up physical therapy at Borgess Fitness Center a month later instead of transferring to a nursing home for rehabilitation. To our amazement and relief, he learned to transfer from wheelchair to regular chair, to walker, to bed, to car, and vice versa and walk with a cane. Since he could no longer drive and Mother was nervous driving in busy traffic, a neighbor drove us to doctor appointments and my home every Sunday afternoon after I spent weekends with my parents in Portage. Brother Paul Belco drove us to church on Saturday vigil masses or on Sundays. As a slender man, he reminded me of a bird flitting around in robes instead of with wings. He spoke in a staccato, high-pitched voice that reverberated throughout the air and buildings. He and his mother often invited us to dinner.

Instead of spending my leisure time swimming, straightening my apartment, and browsing in the public library on weekends, I helped Mom with housecleaning and ironing as well as assisting Dad in independently putting on his shoes and socks to reinforce what he learned in therapy.

Dad's love for us remained steadfast and his upper body strength intact, but his left leg remained paralyzed. Though he spoke coherently, he also lost his mechanical ability which depressed him.

Feeling a strong mental urge to make a trip to Kalamazoo at the spur of the moment a few days before Memorial Day in 2004, Nancy called Mom and Dad to tell them that she and John were coming. After Nancy and John arrived, the five of us drove to South Haven. Dad and John parked on a side street while we ladies shopped at a candle shop and strolled in the streets. Then we went for mass at St. Peter's Catholic Church in Douglas, Michigan, when during the giving of the peace sign, Dad, appearing so very fragile, turned around in the seat to greet the lady behind him. She very gently shook his hand, and a most beatific smile crossed his face as the sun streamed into the church since the weather earlier in the day had been damp and overcast. A choking emotion following a premonition that Dad would not be with us for long overwhelmed me. All day Dad was alert and checking out the countryside, never napping, and enjoying our all being together.

As Nancy helped Dad with his shoes and socks on Sunday morning of that holiday weekend before breakfast, he got John and her aside and told them how he loved both very much.

On June 5, 2004, while Dad and I sat on the patio, enjoying the warm balmy breezes as a harbinger of summer, he gazed at the sky and pensively remarked, "When we die, I wonder if we will recognize our loved ones in heaven. Heaven should be the destination for you girls because you weren't morally or spiritually blind." I interjected, "Dad, according to the Bible, God pities spiritual blindness as well as physical blindness. There is also a Bible verse stating, 'Behold I tell you a mystery. We shall not all sleep, but we shall all be changed in a moment, in the twinkling of an eye at the last trumpet'. Just think, Dad, in heaven you won't have the stroke anymore and I will have perfect vision!" Then I choked up. Seeing tears in my eyes, Dad scolded, "None of that! I want you to brace up! Be strong because your mother will need you!"

He must have had a premonition. Chatting with neighbors sitting in lawn chairs in front of Spring Manor Apartments the next day, Mother asked Dad if he wanted pop, and suddenly he collapsed in his chair. Automatically, I administered CPR, but to my dismay, he did not breathe. Mother stated his face was like a rubber mask. A neighbor called 911.

The Sunday he was stricken, Nancy received such comfort from holding his strong, gnarled fingers all Sunday night at the hospital, listening to his labored breathing via a ventilator. She will never forget the extreme sadness of each day he labored in the hospital, knowing he would never get better and struggling with the wish for him to die quickly to relieve his suffering but hoping he would remain alive for as long as possible. Dad was indeed the rock and the mortar holding our family together.

All week he lay in a coma at Borgess Hospital. Doctors said he had died of another stroke. I shall never forget how the doctors and nurses kept him clean and comfortable, how Brother Paul Belco, Father Larry Farrell, and Father Robert Consani from St. Monica's Church, as well as parishioners and coworkers came to see him in the hospital, and how many people attended his memorial service on June 14 at St. Monica's and graveside service in Alpena on June 15.

At the memorial service, the verses on our Father's Day cards comprised our eulogy for Dad. My verse was:

Daddy's Girl

> My dad is one great reason
> Why I turned out ok.
> He's the guy who taught me
> To stand up and have my say.
> If I could choose from all the dads,
> I'd pick him any day.
> That's why I'm Daddy's Girl.
>
> He's the kind of guy
> Who'll hand you the shirt right off his back.
> He knew the trick of giving me
> The right amount of slack.
> And even if I'd mess things up,
> He wasn't keeping track.
> That's why I'm Daddy's Girl.
>
> Time has changed
> A lot of things.
> But there's one certainty.
> His trust and honest caring
> Guaranteed there'd always be.
> A bond of love and friendship
> Between my dad and me.
> That's why I'm a Daddy's Girl.

Considering his love for baseball and how he supported the Detroit Tigers through thick and thin, my sister Nancy chose a card with a lighter verse which read:
   "Dad, you're like a rare baseball card
One of a kind.
And we wouldn't trade you for anything."
   We both ended, "Dad, Happy Father's Day in heaven!"
   Oh, how we miss him! But loving memories of him captured in these verses will remain forever.
   Dad's death wreaked considerable emotional havoc on Mother who often said losing him meant losing half of herself. Until then, she could not imagine living without him. Therefore, Mother lost interest in many things, including reading, corresponding with friends, and cooking. As Dad had prophesied, she tightly clung to me for support, pleading that I spend every weekend

with her. On one hand, I could have set limits on time spent with Mother, if guilt had not gnawed at me resulting from her explanation to relatives and friends that they moved from Alpena to Portage, Michigan, "so that Sandy wouldn't be alone," never mind my living 30 years on my own. On the other, how would I react to losing a loving, devoted spouse and leaving relatives and many close friends behind in Alpena?

Gradually, I adjusted to a new routine of swimming and doing house cleaning during the evenings after work. Though Mother did make friends with several neighbors encouraging her to participate in some activities, such as crafts, New Year's Eve Bingo/finger-food parties, and Christmas dinners, her attendance was sporadic.

In August, 2005, Mother developed such excruciating pain in both her legs. However, despite medications prescribed by our family doctor, Mother's arthritis became progressively worse to where she had fallen on October 1 and again on October 7, 2007. Though she had in-home physical therapy for a month as recommended by the emergency room physician, Mother lost all her confidence in her ability to live alone, declaring that I must stay with her from then on, because she did not want to go to assisted living or to a nursing home. Hearing that, I attempted to negotiate, "Couldn't you stay in my apartment during the week so I can walk to work? I'll stay with you at Spring Manor on weekends, so you won't have to go to assisted living or a nursing home."

"Take a cab! Since my apartment has its own washer and dryer, I want to stay there and don't want to break the lease."

While her arthritis worsened, Mother's and my independent, fulfilling lives crumbled. Though functioning as an adult caregiver, I rebelled at feeling once again thrust into the adolescent position of kowtowing to Mother's rules while living under her roof, including returning home every workday precisely at 5:30 p.m. for dinner, which caused considerable friction between us. Admiring Mother's strict routine while growing up, because I always had clean clothes ready for school, meals served at regular times, and chores assigned on designated days, I often reacted with exasperation to her inflexibility. Once a vibrant, proud, independent, and athletic person who walked, danced, roller- and ice-skated, tobogganed, and bowled, Mother became increasingly irritated at her inability to perform daily living tasks and flailed at me like a drowning person to a rescuer. Overwhelmed by this new responsibility, I thus doubted my ability as a caregiver.

An unexpected turning point began during the spring of 2008 when driving by Crosstown Parkway Apartments, 550 Crosstown Parkway, in Kalamazoo, we noticed a "Now Leasing" sign for townhomes which Mother had admired. After Nancy and I argued against taking the cab or Care-A-Van to work for the long term, Mother began to realize its inconvenience. Then, Nancy inquired to the manager who informed her that there was a vacant town home apartment available for rent. After Mother moved in on May 12, 2008, how happy I was to resume walking to work during the week and swimming on weekends!

Within these new surroundings, however, Mother's loneliness increased during the day, including frequent telephone calls to me at work. Therefore, my supervisor reprimanded me for poor performance, only allowing Mother to call me during breaks or lunchtime. As time went on, Mother became acquainted with a few neighbors though she did not develop the same rapport with them as she did with the residents at Spring Manor.

Since Mother always wanted us to become strong, independent, self-supporting women, her emotional neediness that emerged since Dad died baffled and annoyed Nancy and me. I often wonder if this stemmed from Mother as a teen taking care of her mother and subsequently losing her to cervical cancer.

Like a child unable to entertain herself, Mother demanded my remaining in the same room with her while she watched TV or napped. If I retreated to another room to read or write letters, she yelled, "Sandy!" raising her voice each time to a higher decibel until I responded. To complete any audio lessons from correspondence courses, read, or listen to music, I waited until Mother went to bed. Ah, the advantage of headphones enabling me to play my portable CD player and talking book machine without disturbing anyone!

Since Mother's arthritis significantly interfered with her cooking and toileting independently during my last year of work, I returned home at lunchtime to assist Mother since she did not want any strangers from home health care agencies in the apartment. Naturally, I missed lunching or exercising with coworkers, but I did what had to be done under these circumstances.

How does one effectively cope with caregiving responsibilities? A former instructor advised me to take each day at a time as a horse walks around with blinders which keep it focused on what is in front of it, preventing it from being scared or distracted.

Prayer aroused serenity as walking, swimming, and listening to music relaxed me. Reading and imagination also provided escape. For instance, during many summer days spent with Mother on the patio, I'd imagined that we both were relaxing and sipping papaya juice on a cruise ship.

Acceptance was a stubborn lock needing WD-40 in adjusting to Mother's numerous wake-up calls for assistance to and from the toilet, Ben Gay rubs, help with keeping bedroom slippers on her feet, and drinks of cold cranberry juice. Ah ha! The tables had turned to where I had become the "parent" and Mom the "child"!

Help springs from inspirational homilies, one of which centered on the theme, "What would Jesus do?" He applied the gentle healing touch to all the ill including the paralytics and lepers with whom he came in contact, lovingly clutching them like lambs to His bosom. He patiently dealt with people's idiosyncrasies, listened, and comforted even if He heard the same complaint a zillion times about an aching back, arm, or a leg. Why didn't I use that more gentle approach as a caregiver?

I also recall another homily expounding on kindness to a father which will not be forgotten, being considerate with him even if his mind should fail and reviling him not in the fullness of one's strength (Wisdom of Ben Sira 3:12-14). As antacid quells the fires of acid reflux, that homily quenched my raging resentment. Hmm! By snapping at Mother when I had to repeat something or when she spilled or dropped things, didn't I revile her for weaknesses that weren't her fault? Thus, reflecting on these homilies gave my attitude toward caregiving a needed face lift.

Something finally clicked after I heard the verse at another mass, "I will lead the blind by ways they have

never known, along unfamiliar paths I will guide them"
(Isaiah 42:16). How I almost missed the opportunity to
be more patient, helpful, and kind to someone else that
caregiving afforded me! My heart changed from that
dark, deep feeling that Mother was a burden to loving
the person for whom I now wished the best.

Reassuring me that I was not alone, my sister, Nancy, as
well as many friends from Kalamazoo Community Chorale who themselves had taken care of aging parents, offered me very much needed support. Besides sending
these people as extensions of Him, God led me to the
following caregiving resources: *Eldercare: Caring for Your
Aging Parents*, authored by Jessica Fagerhaugh and Neil
Griffin as well as Claire Berman's *Caring for Yourself, How
to Help, How to Survive.*

To reiterate, I walked timidly at first and then more
boldly on that caregiving path. In fact, many people have
astonishingly remarked "How interesting! Here you are
visually challenged, yet looking out for someone else,"
since they consider the visually impaired as the ones
needing the care and hence unable to help others. As in
other phases of my life, Mother never allowed me to use
poor vision as an excuse for shirking any responsibility.

Mother and I often teased each other, "Don't we make
a good pair! One of us doesn't see well, and the other
doesn't walk well because of persistent old Arthur!" Yes,
in our situation, each one's strengths compensated for
the other's weaknesses. Since Mother had been around
longer than I, for example, her eyes of wisdom presented a more practical view of life than my own. She helped
me to distinguish people, since her early macular degeneration, a disease blurring central vision as a result
from damage to the macula, a small area at the back of
the eye that helps people see fine details, still did not
yet prevent Mother from recognizing faces. In the fall
of 2011, when Mother's macular degeneration and an
inoperable cataract in the other eye interfered with her
ability to read print, for instance, I introduced Mother to
talking books; large-print check registers; writing, enve-
lope, and signature guides. She embraced the signature,
check writing guides, and large-print check registers but
not talking books since she was hard of hearing and ad-
verse to wearing hearing aids.

Talk about the blind leading the blind (or sighted?) in this incidence! After Dad died, Mother's attempts to drive us to church and grocery shopping unnerved me, because she daydreamed instead of concentrating and drove over the centerline, ignoring incessant horn honking behind us. Once, to my horror, she almost ran into a stop sign. Envisioning air bags striking our faces and dislodging my lens implants, I gasped and hollered, "Stop! Stop!" Apparently, the angels overhead must have guided the steering wheel and her feet to slamming on the brakes–barely a half inch from the stop sign! To my intense relief and to her credit, Mother eventually gave up driving. This decision was safer, proving that I am still alive to write this book.

Rapidly unfolding events during that evening of February 24, 2011, like those surrounding Dad's stroke and death, impressed upon me what little control one has over life's obstructions, detours, and potholes. Neither Mother nor I had foreseen her fall as she tried to get back into bed after I helped her to the toilet at 6:30 p.m. Unable to lift her up by myself, I summoned a neighbor and her girlfriend to assist Mother into bed.

Then around 11:00 p.m. while Mother again called me for assistance in taking her to the bathroom, she complained in slurred speech that she could not walk. When I asked her if she felt numbness in any part of her body, she could not answer. Fearing the possibility of a stroke, I immediately called 911. After the ambulance arrived within a few minutes, off we sped to Borgess Hospital where I stayed all night.

Borgess Hospital ran Mother through a series of tests detecting electrolyte imbalance, urinary tract, and fungal infections which were all working against each other. The physical therapist said the MRI had also revealed a possible (?) small stroke and difficulty swallowing which necessitated her eating pureed food. Mother couldn't walk or raise herself up out of bed or chairs and needed physical therapy for some time. Her heartbeat was irregular, necessitating a pacemaker procedure.

A social worker approached me, gently informing me that physical therapy administered at the hospital was insufficient due to Mother's weakness; therefore, she would need more therapy in a rehab facility or nursing home. "Oh, God, no!" I cried, "Mother made my sister and me promise never to put her into any nursing homes, since she abhors them."

Laughing wryly, he asked, "Well, isn't that a rather dangerous promise?" He suggested I read some literature that he offered me on rehabilitation facilities in Kalamazoo, choose three over the weekend, and then he and my family would discuss this on Monday. He recommended Borgess Gardens as the newest and closest to Borgess Hospital. John took Nancy and me to tour three facilities on Sunday.

Since Mother was transferred on Monday from Intensive Care Unit to Borgess Heart Center section of the hospital, much to our initial disappointment, we were assigned to another social worker who reviewed our choices of rehabilitation facilities and telephoned Sister Tammy, Entrance and Discharge Director, at Borgess Gardens to inquire if there were any beds available. Since four discharges were scheduled at the end of the week, the social worker-initiated paperwork, and we then investigated Borgess Gardens.

Borgess Gardens' teal and beige lobby contained a library, a computer, several easy chairs, and tables. The brown-and white wallpapered dining rooms with brown tablecloth-covered tables appeared spotless. The chapel as well as the hallway walls decorated in cream and beige wallpaper and floors covered with cinnamon carpet except for main ones tiled in teal and beige leaves aroused serenity.

Unlike other nursing facilities Nancy and I have visited, no urine or fecal odors assailed us as we walked in the door. Sister Tammy went over the paperwork previously completed, and Mother's room would be ready when she arrived—H-12 in Heirloom Garden. The main building was divided into four sections or "gardens": Heirloom, Flower, Enchanted, and Tea Garden, each distinguished by its own planter of specific flowers.

Following a successful pacemaker surgery the day before, Mother's afternoon transfer from Borgess Hospital to Borgess Gardens on Friday, March 4, 2011, did not happen as seamlessly as Nancy and I had anticipated. Contrary to what we had expected upon admitting Mother to Borgess Gardens, we did not receive any explanation of staff responsibilities, patient menus, establishment of a therapy program, and resident preparedness. Upon Mother's transfer from Borgess Hospital, the personal care assistants were unaware of the extent of her lack of mobility, not knowing whether one or two assistants were required. With the help of Lifeline, they transferred Mother to a wheelchair with two different size footrests which were too long for her. We were uncertain regarding whether she would be placed on a puréed or a general diet and were told we would have to wait until Monday for a speech therapist's evaluation. Unaware that there was only a skeleton staff on the weekends, we obtained information piecemeal.

Another frustrating case in point was the dining room situation. Mother had difficulty eating but liked the social contact with the two ladies she had met in the Pines dining room. However, on Monday March 7, we were informed that because she needed assistance in eating, she was transferred to the Oaks dining room where she had little social contact. Later, we discovered that people only certified in feeding were working in that dining room.

Though by accident we ran into the dietitian who met with Mother about her dietary preferences, we were informed that the speech therapist wasn't planning to see Mother until Wednesday. Intervening, the dietitian performed the swallowing evaluation on Mother early Monday afternoon. We did not know until the activity director mentioned while inventorying Mom's interests that there would be a therapy progress meeting including the physical therapist, occupational therapist, nurses, and social worker on Thursday, March 10, regarding a plan for Mom's stay. Following the progress meeting, Mother's plan finally fell into place.

To develop eye/hand coordination and strength, Mother underwent therapeutic exercises which involved card matching, clothespin tree, raising popsicle-shaped dowels as high as possible, throwing beanbags into baskets placed at varying distances. Therapy also included placing plastic Thera bands under Mother's legs, holding up the ends with her lifting and swinging her legs, increasing the resistance and the number of lifts per day. Mother also worked on self-care skills such as washing her face, brushing teeth, applying makeup, combing her hair, and dressing independently with a cardboard sock aid by placing the socks over the cardboard, and pulling the straps to put the sock on the foot.

Initially, Mother's weakness impeded her progress. Finally, within the first month, she could transfer from the wheelchair to grab bars in the bathroom to hoist herself up for someone to pull on her underpants and slacks. During the tenth week of therapy, therapists also showed her how to get into bed and into a car. Within the last two weeks, she concentrated on walking various distances in the building and walking on a wide wooden beam while grabbing on bars to the sides to maintain balance.

Therapists also attempted to improve Mother's range of motion through a windshield wiper exercise on a half-moon shaped device on which Mother moved a lever at different motions, gradually sweeping in wider arcs. Despite ultrasound treatments, arthritic pain still hampered Mother's progress as did Mother's unwillingness to learn how to apply makeup herself, despite occupational therapists' insistence to be released from Borgess Gardens.

No matter how attractive the buildings or pleasant the staff, nursing facilities are depressing places associated with people broken in body, mind, and spirit. In fact, many Borgess Garden's residents sitting at dinner or in wheelchairs by the aviaries or aquarium did not talk. No doubt, they formerly told captivating stories sadly obscured by Alzheimer's disease. For example, an English resident remembered working as a shoe salesperson while living in London during the Blitz but could not recall her family home or her siblings' names. Therefore, I often worried about how the surroundings affected Mother, because she was so unhappy there, unable to enjoy bantering with these residents as she once did with neighbors and party guests.

Borgess Gardens had beautiful aviaries resembling huge china closets made of glass panes supported by wooden panels but consisting of ivy and straw lining the back wall of the aviaries from roof to floor, perches fastened to the wall, a fluorescent light in the center of the aviary. Straw nests bordered the top of the aviary bustling with blue-gray doves, zebra finches, and society finches. Blue cap waxbills perched with their tail feathers facing me. How happy I was to see the birds up close as they flitted from perch to nest, courted while chasing each other, fed from a dish at the bottom of the aviary but drank water by pecking at metal cups with their beaks activating a pumping mechanism inside a box to prevent harmful bacteria from multiplying in stagnant water placed in a dish!

However, Nancy reacted with profound sadness while she observed the birds in the aviary as they reminded her of the residents trapped in their broken bodies. This analogy could also apply to blind people confined to asylums which, though sheltering them, deprived them of their freedom and dignity.

Like newly blinded students attending the Center, Mother had her own difficulties adjusting to the Borgess Garden's routine, insisting that aides put her pajamas on at 4:30 p.m. as I did at home or that she go to bed at 6:30 p.m. regardless of whether aides were still serving dinner trays to other residents. Being away from home distressed Mother.

Finally, she was discharged on Good Friday, April 22, 2011. Mother was barely home a month when on May 19, Mary Ruczynski, our cousin, called, informing us that our uncle Leonard, Mother's only surviving brother of the three, died after frequent bouts of pneumonia. While we attended the funeral on Memorial Day weekend, relatives marveled that Mother's physical strength would enable her to travel.

Spending a week from June 25-July 2, 2011, with Nancy and John in Carmel, Indiana, afforded Mother and me a needed change of scenery from daily caregiving. We attended a jazz concert and visited the town of French Lick known for West Baden Springs Resort in which the notorious and the renowned, including Al Capone and Helen Keller, stayed to be rejuvenated by its mud and sulfur baths. Chris Bundy's *West Baden Springs: Legacy of Dreams* excellently chronicles the history of West Baden Springs.

However, the remainder of the summer was not blissful, since Mother launched into many tirades about my leaving her alone when I swam and sang in the Kalamazoo Community Chorale. Keeping the peace but also especially missing the exhilaration of learning new music, performing in Christmas, spring concerts, and in Chorale banquet talent shows, I regretfully quit Chorale while caring for Mom. One cannot turn off thirty-year friendships like a faucet.

Deathly afraid to sleep alone in her bedroom, even though I was right there with her in her apartment, Mother slept in a dining room chair.

Again, on August 21, 2011, Mother fell while I assisted her to the toilet. Another harrowing ambulance ride to Borgess Hospital ensued where Mother was admitted for dehydration and urinary tract infection with the recommendation by Borgess physicians for some stamina buildup before returning to her apartment. After investigating rehabilitation facilities, Nancy and I decided on Friendship Village where Mother was transferred on Wednesday, August 24.

Like therapists at Borgess Gardens, Mother's therapist at Friendship Village involved me in hands-on demonstration of all exercises and created large-print copies of exercises as a reference which would enable me to practice with Mother at home. Oh, what a struggle! Whether Mom's lack of progress in therapy here resulted from her inability to process information or from stubbornness was difficult to determine. Longing to return home, Mother did not want to be at Friendship Village any more than she wanted to be at Borgess Gardens. Following the care conference, Mother returned home on September 29, 2011, to attempt follow-up in-home therapy from Great Lakes Home Care and Hospice.

During October and November, Mother resented the continuous invasion of therapists in her home. Though walking remained difficult, at least she pivoted to the toilet and chairs. However, afraid of falling and preferring to sit all day and sleep in her dining room chair, she refused to sleep in bed and further therapy that would help her get in and out of bed. Sitting in one place resulted in bedsores.

As time went on, a fiend appeared to snatch Mother's personality from her body, replacing it with that of a stranger akin to the possessed girl in the movie, *The Exorcist*. When Mother hurled into her "Help me!" outbursts, she abruptly changed from her usually pleasant, well-modulated voice into a raspy, crackling one. This terrified me as well as her calling for dead people she knew such as her mother, Uncle Joe, Dad, Uncle Frank, and Uncle Leonard. From Thanksgiving to December 11, Mother woke me up every five to ten minutes, demanding help to the bathroom even though she could not void, drinks of cranberry juice and applications of Ben Gay to her sore shoulder. Unable to get sufficient rest, both of us woke up tired and frazzled the next day. I, too, became increasingly irritable due to sleeplessness and Mother's inability to understand my need for rest.

On December 11 when I helped Mother to the toilet, she fell wedged between the toilet and the wall. I called Lifeline, and again Mother was admitted to Borgess Hospital for dehydration and electrolyte imbalance and diagnosed with a slight crack in her left foot. Upon Dr. Oprescu's recommendation for more therapy before returning home, Nancy and I chose the Springs at 1451 Bronson Way in Kalamazoo. Being a smaller facility with 41 patients, hopefully the staff would give Mother more prompt one-on-one care, but "Same song, third verse, a little bit louder and a little bit worse!" typified Mother's reaction to the daily routine and therapy at the Springs.

After four weeks passed, to our dismay, the Springs staff informed Nancy and me that time was running out on Medicare payments due to Mother's poor progress in therapy. On Tuesday, January 24, 2012, Mother was scheduled for a home evaluation to see how she could navigate around her apartment with a wheelchair. This was recommended as safer than walking with a walker. Confronted with the possibility of placing Mother into long-term care or assisted living if further therapy proved futile, Nancy delved into required eligibility qualifications for Medicaid and assisted living and long-term care facilities that would accept Medicaid patients.

Mother passed her home evaluation with flying colors. In the meantime, the therapist taught me how to assist Mother in transferring from the wheelchair to toilet and wheelchair to walker to bed and vice versa, guiding Mother by holding on to a gait belt fastened on her waist. How happy we were when informed that Mother would be discharged on Friday, February 3, with recommendations for home therapy with Great Lakes Home Care and Hospice!

However, our relief was short-lived. Though her pulse-ox readings ranged anywhere from 90 to 97%, Mother insisted that she still needed oxygen. Naturally, her discharge filled us with apprehension instead of joy. At the beginning of the week, Mother sporadically hyperventilated and occasionally asked me to open the patio door despite freezing temperatures so she could breathe better. At night, she begged me to sleep with her in the living room as she was afraid to be left alone. By the end of that week, both my alarm and temper reached their zenith. In fact, I wonder how I mustered all necessary restraint to avoid clobbering her with her wheelchair footrests.

At 4:30 on Sunday morning, February 12, I woke to the horrendous screams of Mother crying out between labored gasps that she could not breathe and that she was dying. Following our hair-raising ambulance ride to Borgess Hospital, I made sure that Mother was settled comfortably as possible. As soon as my sister arrived at the hospital, she and I then spent most of the day consulting with what seemed to be almost every medical professional on staff from a cardiologist to a gerontologist. Upon admission and thorough examination, doctors stated that Mother had fluid buildup in her lungs due to congestive heart failure.

Dr. Jeanette Meyer, an internist specializing in geriatrics and palliative care, warned us, "I know the goal is for your mother to go home after therapy. Chances are also great she may not go home after the 50 days. Due to her irregular heartbeat and congestive heart failure, resuscitating her would be more harmful with broken ribs, and tubes. She does have dementia which will also get worse as time goes by." This was the first time that any doctors have ever confronted us with a diagnosis like that. Dr. Shiree stated that Mother's heart was functioning at 30-35% according to the most recent ECHO. They were preparing us for the possibility of her long-term care if therapy did not prove successful. Dr. Shiree recommended several weeks of physical therapy to regain Mother's strength. Since a bed was available at Borgess Gardens, she was transferred there on February 16 from Borgess Hospital.

Attempting to allay any unpleasant surprises arising from an upcoming care conference scheduled within two weeks, the nursing supervisor cautioned me that mother's medical condition "had reached the point where she needs more care than you are able to give." Nancy and I had to accept the inevitable.

During the care conference on March 1, the nursing supervisor informed us that medically, she had many scruples against discharging Mother to home both for her safety and mine. Therefore, she recommended that Mother remain at Borgess Gardens for long-term care. Though medically fragile and in need of 24-hour nursing care, Mother was nowhere near the point of hospice care.

The nursing supervisor's recommendation finally allayed Nancy's and my concerns regarding my increasing burnout and Mother's potential loss of her place at Borgess Gardens if she stayed at home for only a week or a month following her discharge, then returned to the hospital, and subsequently were placed in a substandard facility. Neither would home respite care be a viable option, given its exclusion from Medicaid coverage and Mother's antagonism toward home health care aides.

Mother reacted to the news with a welter of emotions: shock, disappointment, dismay, sorrow, denial, and rage, lamenting, "It's too bad you save so much all of your life and then end up spending down everything that you have to $2,000 to qualify for Medicaid!" and "You mean I will never get out of here? I could just cry!" Then, unlike her stoical nature, Mother did sob. Hearing her sobs ripped Nancy's and my hearts to ribbons. Despite their reassurance of their best care, the staff could not console Mother. Though I intellectually grasped the Medicaid spend-down requirements, emotionally, remorse plagued me as if I were an accomplice in an unspeakable crime, divesting Mother of her assets.

To cheer Mother, I decorated her room with silk-flowered wreaths and arrangements from her apartment plus all the cards from relatives and friends. Mom's room overlooked a garden filled with seasonal grasses, pink peonies, and other beds of annual flowers. I shall never forget how beautiful the setting was.

How daunting the tasks that lay ahead in the upcoming months for Nancy and me! We had to obtain the surrender values of life insurance policies, cash in on CD's and savings accounts, set up an irrevocable trust for Mom's prepaid funeral expenses before applying for Medicaid, revoke Mother's lease on her apartment, empty my apartment of my furniture for donations to NuWay to make room for furniture Mother wanted me to have, and move that into my apartment. Though a few months before, I had applied to take over Mother's apartment since it was a cozy apartment on one floor, with a patio, its own washer and dryer, my application was rejected, because my income exceeded the guidelines stipulated by Housing and Urban Development for residents living in government subsidized housing at Crosstown Parkway Apartments. I, too, grappled with hypertension, cervical polyps, and slightly elevated blood sugar diagnosed during an annual physical as well as adjusting to a low-sodium, sugar-free diet. A gynecologist to whom my primary care physician had referred me for follow-up recommended outpatient surgery scheduled for May 22, 2012. Darn it! One thing after another!

Dragging on, Lent prompted me to reflect on Jesus' slow agonizing death on the cross and offer tribulations as a sacrifice. Two weeks before Easter, while listening to a priest's homily illustrating the Good Fridays of tribulation and Easter Sundays of triumph in our lives, I saw the humorous side of it as a curious analogy to eggs. "How do you like your Good Fridays: hard-boiled, scrambled, over-easy, or sunny-side up?" This was reminiscent of childhood lunchtime egg-salad sandwiches and scrambled eggs as substitutions for meat.

Easter weekend finally arrived when we brought Mother home via Metro County Connect on Saturday, April 7, and had a beautiful, scrumptious Easter ham dinner from Ample Pantry and a relaxing time opening gifts and gazing at Easter decorations I had made. Easter Sunday mass hymns reverberated with glory.

Finally gaining our second wind, Nancy, John, and I donated my unneeded furniture, books, wall hangings, and CD's to NuWay and then scheduled an appointment with Two Men and a Truck to transfer Mother's furniture from her apartment into mine. Mother and I also wrote a letter to her apartment manager revoking her lease.

How does one deal with a parent in denial, believing that she would return home someday even though we realized that Mother could not? On lucid days, she knew why I was moving back to my own apartment. One day, she asked me, "If Borgess Gardens discharges me, can I live with you?" I replied, "Yes, if they discharge you. Right now, they will not if you can't walk."

When I did remind her that Borgess Gardens would be her permanent home, Mother became very agitated. Promising her that she would return home when she could not to build up her hopes would be unfair to her. Brother Paul's comforting words, "I know you are doing this with all of your loving care, and you can hold your heads up high," assuaged any unwarranted guilt arising from Mom's attitude of childlike selfishness. Boxed into a corner with no exit, I was haunted by the specter of Mother's ever-lingering illness. How many more eight- to ten-hour daily vigils at Borgess Gardens and Mother's agonizing shrieks upon my daily leaving could I endure without losing my health and sanity?

Meanwhile, the "Creating Confident Caregivers" course offered by our local health department spared me from implosion. Support and brainstorming that sprang from emotional venting among classmates provided me with objective solutions to problems and more inner strength and confidence. Soon, I realized why Mother was no longer interested in TV, because the news anchors' continuous verbiage mentally overwhelmed her. After the instructor explained how repeatedly driving her in her wheelchair and answering questions comforted Mother, I stopped scolding Mother when she asked repetitive questions and insisted that I constantly wheel her around Borgess Gardens. Had I completed this course a few years earlier, I would have taken her strange behavior more in stride.

The possibility of dementia never crossed my mind until doctors at Borgess Hospital and the nurse practitioner at Borgess Gardens confirmed its diagnosis. Until then, how I missed the signs! Initially, I did notice her increasing irritability and agitation after Mother moved from Spring Manor Apartments to Crosstown Parkway Apartments which I construed as bitterness at moving. Soon after, she needed more help with balancing her checkbook and paying bills, lashed out at John, Nancy, and me for no apparent reason, uncharacteristically ridiculed my need for further education, and accused cab drivers of taking me into the woods and raping me when I returned late from grocery shopping. When she no longer could make important decisions for herself, Nancy and I signed paperwork relating to hospitalization and therapy. Thank God, our parents had the foresight years ago to write a will designating durable powers of attorney!

All afternoon and evening on Monday, May 14, Mother also behaved erratically. At the dentist's office, she yelled, "Sandy, help me! Why are you taking so long?" as if a tape recording were continually playing inside of her. While comforting her, the receptionist explained that I was having my teeth cleaned. As we passed Borgess Hospital upon her return to Borgess Gardens, Mother demanded, "Don't take me to Borgess Hospital. I don't want to go there!" The Pride Ambulance driver reassured Mother that she was taking her back to Borgess Gardens. Arriving in the parking lot, Mother pleaded, "Please don't take me back here! I beg you! I hate it here!" I gently reminded Mother that Borgess Gardens was now her home, not Crosstown Parkway Apartments, since her medical condition rendered her to be unsafe living independently. That evening, Mother bellowed, "Help me, Sandy! Come on, Sandy!" until she was sedated.

Finally realizing that she would never return home to Crosstown Parkway Apartments, Mother might have given up as a result. Eventually, from May 15 until May 18, Mother gradually faded, sleeping longer in her wheelchair during the day and only passively attending birthday parties and musical programs or going outside. Visiting Mother on Friday, May 18, I was dismayed to find her in bed. Following the Borgess Gardens' staff recommendations to let her rest, I prayed at Nazareth Holy Family Chapel for Mother and my upcoming cervical polyp surgery and D&C on May 22, 2012, which turned out fine. Prayer gave me that much needed serenity of being comforted in Jesus' arms.

On Saturday morning, May 19, Mother slept in her wheelchair. To our alarm at lunchtime, the aids could not arouse her and instructed me to take her to the nurse who informed me that, suspecting she had a urinary tract infection the night before, they took a urine analysis. During the afternoon, Mom woke up, hollering

"Suzy!" and speaking in gibberish. In the meantime, lab results confirmed a urinary tract infection of 700 white blood cell count! Normally the count was slightly over 100. Mother remained in bed several more days with a high fever.

During a May 24th conference with Nancy and me, the nurse practitioner and the Borgess Gardens chaplain informed us that Mother's medical condition reached the point where she needed hospice care, giving her possibly one week to live at the most. Imagine being hit with that devastating news!

From Friday the 25th to Sunday, May 27th, Mother somewhat rallied, sipping ginger ale from a small plastic cup, or some chicken broth and eating applesauce, chocolate pie and vanilla ice cream mixed with chopped Dove chocolate caramels which she enjoyed. Due to the Memorial Day holiday, Hospice nurses did not arrive until Tuesday, May 29.

On May 29, Mother appeared more contented than I had ever seen her. One of the aides gave her a sponge bath, then powered and sprayed her with Wings perfume and dressed her in a clean hospital gown. Surrounded by Nancy and me, she received the attention she enjoyed and was even laughing. That image of her we will always remember and cherish.

During the following days, Mother's breathing became more labored.' Since she became so weak, she could no longer kiss us on the lips, and her "I love you's" became fainter. To calm her, the chaplain brought in a CD player and played relaxing classical and 1940s music, and we sang "I Love You a Bushel and a Peck," "Cheek to Cheek," and "Sentimental Journey." Sisters, a chaplain from St. Augustine, and Father Farrell from St. Monica's Parish gave her the anointing of the sick and other blessings.

Nancy had a little cheer which she either began or ended a phone conversation to Mom; "Who's the best Mom in the world?" and Mom would say "Me!" Nancy cried "Louder!" and Mom then said, "I am." Mom was able to answer faintly until Wednesday, May 30, when she did not respond to our voices.

On Friday afternoon, June 1, after Nancy and I left Mother's room for a brief break and returned there a half an hour later, Nancy noticed Mother not breathing. One of the nurses came in, checked Mother's vitals, and sobbed, "Virginia has gone to the Lord!" Sadness, disbelief, and numbness swept over us as we bade her goodbye and packed her belongings. Ironically, two weeks before, we had made prepaid arrangements for Mother to preserve assets for funeral expenses needed before applying for Medicaid. Another irony struck me: While the nurses attended to Mom and we grieved, the men outside washing windows were oblivious to the patient dying inside her room. The reality of now being adult orphans penetrated our hearts like a clasp knife.

As an uplifting celebration of Mother's life and transition into resurrection, the funeral mass highlighted the themes in readings from Wisdom 3:1 "The souls are in the hand of God and no torment shall touch them"; Romans 6:4 "Just as Christ was raised from the dead by the glory of the Father, we, too, might live in the newness of life" and from John 14:2 "In my Father's house are many dwelling places...And if I go to prepare a place for you, I will come back again and take you to myself." Sunlight shined through the stain-glass windows creating dazzling images depicting Bible stories in brilliant cobalt blue, topaz, emerald, and red-orange colors. Like an angel, the cantor sang Schubert's "Ave Maria" and "Be Not Afraid", "I am the Bread of Life", "On Eagle's Wings", and How Great Thou Art" as she led the congregation through these songs we had requested. What a glimpse of heaven we received that day!

Following Father McCallum's excellent homily epitomizing Mother, Nancy and I also presented eulogies of her. Whereas mine praised her impeccable dress and mouth-watering meals and desserts, Nancy's portrayed the themes of faith, security, and love Mom instilled in her as she described her reactions to Mother's leaving after surgery for strabismus at Harper Hospital in Detroit, a classmate's mother's death, and learning to drive. After the mass, we hosted the guests to a delicious luncheon at Holiday Inn.

Emotionally, that year, Nancy, John, and I gradually moved onward and healed with Nancy enrolling in bible study/genealogy classes, library volunteering, and participating in parish ministry while I returned to taking Hadley Correspondence Courses and singing in the Kalamazoo Community Chorale. Meanwhile, I began bible study, singing in church choir, and volunteering at Borgess Gardens and Friendship Village. Possible activities included helping residents at Bingo and in making bracelets, card playing and visiting, contributing to bake sales, and participating in talent shows. I shall always be close to my sister and brother-in-law. God willing, we shall overcome!

CHAPTER 13: RETIREMENT OR REFOCUSING?

Retirement evokes diverse images and lifestyles: sunny beaches in Florida or Hawaii, endless rounds of golf, or sitting in a rocking chair watching the world go by. Not for me! I would only sit in a rocker if it had a high-performance engine and racing slicks. Vroom! Vroom! On the contrary, I anticipated senior field trips to museums, concerts, plays in Stratford, Ontario, auditing courses at Western Michigan University, countless hours of swimming, attending health seminars at Borgess Medical Center, religious retreats, conferences, and Bible study at church.

I also planned to work until I was 65; however, Michigan had other ideas for its baby-boomer state employees, due to its ballooning budget deficit. Like the Godfather, Governor Jennifer Granholm presented an offer we could not refuse: early retirement eligibility for state employees aged 55 and over who had worked for 25 years or aged 60 who had worked for ten years. Being 61 years of age and having worked for nearly 37 years at the Michigan Commission for the Blind Training Center, I certainly qualified for early retirement though I was initially sad about doing so, having always looked forward to working every day. Considering the usual summer deluge of high school and college students receiving training at the Center which then resulted in the heaviest staff workloads, I waited to retire until September 1, 2010.

Following two months of intensive planning and preparation, the staff and my family threw me a most memorable retirement party during the afternoon of September 24, 2010. Since I wanted something different from the most pre-

viously prevalent potlucks and dinner parties at restaurants in which guests either had to bring dishes to pass
or pay for their own meals, my family had purchased attractive vegetable and fruit trays, turkey, beef, and ham
sandwich platters, barbecued meatballs, and a beautiful
sheet cake made of two white battered layers filled with
Bavarian cream and decorated with white frosting and
gold, turquoise, and purple letters, "Congratulations, on
your retirement, Sandy Fortier," which color coordinated with the retirement banners, helium balloons, paper
napkins, plates, and cups on the tables and raffle tickets
for a door prize.

The dietary staff made refreshing ginger ale and grape
juice punch and furnished all the tablecloths, coffee
pot, and punch bowl.

As the table displayed diverse plates of delectable finger foods, the program presented a variety of clever,
heart-warming, and funny speeches. Though I enjoyed
them all, I will include the most salient ones here.

"Sandy Fortier
S: is for Sagacious because sagacious means wise, clever, perceptive, erudite, astute, and knowledgeable. S is
also for Sweet because Sandy is Sweet. But most of all,
S is for Successful, because Sandy has overcome many
challenges to be Successful.

A: is for Always and Attitude and Active because Sandy
Always has a great Attitude. And she Always participates
in a lot of Activities. But most importantly, Sandy Always
brings lots of great treats to eat.

N: is for Nice and Noble and Naughty. We all know
that Sandy is Nice and Noble. But some of us know that
Sandy can be just a little bit Naughty. We've partied with
her and watched her at state staff meetings.

D: is for Dutiful and Delicious. Sandy always attends to
her Duties Dutifully. She also Dutifully makes Delicious
treats for us to eat.

Y: is for Youthful because Sandy hasn't aged a bit in 37
years. And Y is for You because we love You.

F: is for Faithful, Friend, and Food. Sandy is a Faithful
Friend who always makes Fine Food For her Friends.

O: is for On-Key because Sandy always gets the staff to
sing Happy Birthday On-Key.

R: is for Religious, Respectful, and Rowdy. Sandy has a deep Religious faith, and she is always Respectful of everybody, But Sandy can also be Rowdy. Remember some of those volleyball parties and the picnics?

T: is Tenacious because Sandy never gives up. Sandy Tenaciously bugs us to get those progress reports in, sometimes even after we've sent them.

I: is for Individual, and Independent, and Intellect, because Sandy is a unique Individual with an Independent Intellect that never quits,

E: is for Eager because Sandy is always Eager to do her share, especially when it comes to making something great to Eat, another E word.

R: is Retired and Retirement because Sandy after 37 wonderful years, you are now officially Retired, and we all hope you enjoy your well-deserved Retirement. YOU GO GIRL!"

Nancy Fezzey's Retirement Speech for Sandra Fortier: "Thank you for being here to celebrate Sandy. I thank God and Mom and Dad for giving me the best sister I could ever have. Sandy is a kind-hearted, giving person who never runs from a challenge nor reneges on her commitments.

Her love of music began in her Teeter Babe amazing all who heard her hum to the radio—a prelude to her long-time participation in the Kalamazoo Community Chorale.

With the support of progressive parents, she excelled in a school system ill-equipped at the time to deal with special needs. Sandy mastered a bike, bowling, and swimming. There wasn't a daring-do ride at the county fair she wouldn't try much to her sister's chagrin.

She even signed up for driver's ed and would have rivaled Helio Castroneves had she had a bit more vision!

As a child, Sis instigated exploration of mysterious old buildings—even a forbidden antique shop!

Being a twin is a wonderful experience—a special bond and has been a good "journey".

Sandy, Mother, John, and I salute you and wish you many joys in your retirement.

I know Dad is in heaven smiling down on you. You are loved very much."

Despite her arthritis afflicting her from 2005 when I was still working until the rest of her life, Mother marched up to the podium to give a heartwarming speech regarding how she and Dad never considered me as handicapped and that I attended regular classes all through school. She included humorous stories, one about Nancy and my sleeping in our own cribs due to my constant kicking and wiggling. The other described her exclamation of "Holy Moses!" when we performed well on the potty and our telling her, "We have to make Holy Moses," until we learned the correct words for going to the bathroom. That elicited many chuckles.

A choir of coworkers performed this song to the tune of "Mother."

S-A-N-D-R–A

S is for the Smiles she always gave us
A is for All the love she brings
N is for the Noshes that she made us
D is for the Dandy way she sings
*   (the way she sings)*
R is for Reports she's always after
A she is like an Angel without wings
(without the wings)
Put them altogether, they spell SANDRA
A name that is heart of MCB.

The program was spectacular enough but how surprised I was to receive a DVD player, and $500! How could these 37 years result in this culmination without God's design and direction, as well as the ardent support of my co-workers, and family, the best gifts of all? I felt both proud and humbled.

Reflecting upon my rewarding career as a word processing assistant, eventually I realized that doing what satisfied me and how God's and my self-perceptions were more important than others' perceptions of me, prestige, or title. In 1971 and for a long time after that, Mother, and I both had handled ourselves very badly by regarding my student teaching as a shameful event instead of a learning experience on relating to people and knowing oneself. How silly that was! Teaching was not my niche after all.

As time went on, I met former classmates and other people in my workplace who have changed careers. Perhaps what I have done might never have been as prestigious in Mother's eyes as elementary school or rehabilitation teaching would have been, yet I enjoyed secretarial work more than teaching and steadfastly dedicated myself to it. Joining Professional Secretaries International (later renamed International Association of Administrative Professionals), I crusaded with other secretaries to elevate the profession to the status it deserves.

Other reflections sparked another insight about blindness within me of which the visually challenged have an advantage over the sighted in that since they can't always see how others react to their actions, they look within themselves to see what sits well with their values and standards. Like pinball machines, sighted people change how they act to fit how others respond the way a pinball bounces from one station to another.

The first two years of retirement meant downsizing expectations. Instead of experiencing anticipated pleasure-filled days of senior bus trips, Bible study, volunteering, or auditing courses at Western Michigan University, I initially became disillusioned, because care-giving responsibilities described in the previous chapter thwarted these expectations. Now so much wiser in knowing that caregiving is a full-time job, I can see that I had no other alternative than putting these other pursuits on the back burner during that phase.

Thereafter, memories of our family's emotional trauma after Mother's death impelled me to maintain good health by eating properly and exercising. Furthermore, I have resumed calisthenics, walking, and swimming four to five times a week. Exercising and following the low-sodium, sugar-free diet have been difficult but must be done to maintain glucose and blood pressure at normal levels, thereby decreasing my chances of complications, such as total blindness, kidney failure, foot problems, and dental disease, developing over time from diabetes diagnosed in February, 2015.

Reading inspirational books about people with disabilities, celebrities, and Holocaust survivors has occupied much of my time. Moreover, I have kindled a dormant interest in American and English literature since I left college. Wisdom which comes with maturity enables me to derive deeper meaning from the authors' messages in poetry and prose through required reading in the Carmel Public Library book club as well as independent recreational reading.

How could I become a more impassioned Catholic? I must admit a yearning for a more intimate relationship with Jesus, God the Father, and the Holy Spirit. Since the priests I have known while growing up appeared so austere and distant, I dismissed God as being the same way. In fact, I even pictured Him as an unforgiving God relentlessly ferreting out sinners much as an Orkin exterminator shining his flashlight on cockroaches and gleefully zapping them.

However, the Holy Spirit's prodding to attend a Dynamic Catholic seminar held at our parish during the summer of 2013, reading Matthew Kelly's *The Four Signs of a Dynamic Catholic*, and participating in a Dynamic Catholic group became a game changer for me in devoting a scheduled intimate prayer time each day, delving into Old and New Testament Scripture, and, upon the group's invitation, attending a pilgrimage regarding the Passion of Jesus Christ in St. John's, Indiana. I felt as if I were transported back 2000 years to Jerusalem with 40 bronze life-size figures and landscaped gardens replicating the Holy Land. Touching the statues including the wounds inflicted upon Jesus hanging on the cross and being able to walk up to the bronze soldiers and feel their sneering facial expressions filled me with such an intense poignancy and repentance.

Through Lectio Divina, a process of praying with the Scriptures that promotes union with the living God, involving reading, reflecting on words which captured our attention during the reading, prayerfully responding to words Jesus spoke, and then focusing our attention completely on God in loving adoration, I've taken similar journeys back 2000 years from books of Genesis to Paul's letters. I no longer regarded the Bible as an old fossil. Considering similarities of human nature and social problems then and now and what we could learn from God's teachings opened many floodgates of meaning. Scripture finally came alive!

Hence Holy Spirit filled members of this Dynamic Catholic Group encouraged me to fulfill Matthew Kelly's characteristics of a vibrant Catholic by assuming various roles as an anchor, an inspirer, and a nurturer. They specifically included being a steadfast friend and confident, facilitating a Bible study lesson, functioning as a reliable friendly visitor and activities assistant in Bingo, crafts, talent shows, and singalongs at nursing facilities as well as other community service projects which involved assembling personal care packages for people undergoing drug rehabilitation, hospice dwellings, Ministry with Community, and St. Vincent de Paul. I still needed to work on evangelization, which is the most difficult for me to embrace; because while growing up, I always thought that religion was a private aspect of one's life. I wished to evangelize without resorting to high-pressure tactics.

So, for the past several years, I continued a comfortable, fulfilling routine of swimming, Kalamazoo Community Chorale, volunteering at Friendship Village, Borgess Gardens, church choir and Dynamic Catholic group projects, and Bible study, never foreseeing what would careen around the cul-de-sac.

It crashed into me around the end of July, 2017, when my apartment manager notified all tenants that the present owners were eventually looking to sell the complex; and that all tenants would have to sign a lease to protect them against indiscriminate eviction or increased rent. I railed, "Where was God?" Either the owners would completely renovate the apartment complex or allow it to deteriorate since the building was 70 years old with an antiquated boiler. Somehow this made no sense though I knew like a loving parent God wants the best for us and never leaves anything to chance.

Where would I stay if my apartment were renovated or move if the new owners were to raze the complex? No telling what they would have in mind.

In the meantime, my sister's, and brother–in–law's more frequent reminders of our "not getting any younger" and a friend's Holy Spirit filled advice, "When you get older, it is more important to be near family since you have no family near you. Nancy and John also may not be able to make the drive to your place in the future, either. "God's help and some deep, silent discernment will lead the way and open all of the doors," persuaded

me to move closer to them in Carmel, Indiana. Shortly after I informed Nancy and John of my decision regarding the move, they set up appointments for me to
meet with Prime Life Enrichment, an activity center for
seniors 50 years and older, and managers at senior apartments in August, 2017. Preferring Rosewalk on Main
because it was immaculately maintained and centrally
located within walking distance of downtown Carmel, I
placed my name on a waiting list—and the long wait for
a vacancy began. God's testing of our patience was finally rewarded two days after Christmas when the manager
of Rosewalk called me at home in Kalamazoo, informing me of a vacant second-floor, one-bedroom apartment with a courtyard view and comfortable patio with
shed for additional storage. Following my sister's and
brother-in-law's inspection and glowing approval, I
moved in at the end of February 2018.

Soon, I became acclimated to my new surroundings,
including participating in a non-denominational neighborhood Bible study group and library book club, exploring downtown Carmel, lap swimming at Monon
Center, attending exercise classes and lunch/learn programs running the gamut from a musician performing
with spoons to topics on fire safety and preventing Medicare fraud at Prime Life Enrichment, becoming a pa-
rishioner at St. Louis de Montfort, and volunteering as a
friendly visitor at Manor Care of Summer Trace.

Unfamiliar with roundabouts during the first time I
had ventured into downtown Carmel, I stood on their
medians, waiting for traffic to stop while waiting to cross
streets. Naturally, Nancy and John reacted with alarm
when I related this exploit, "You did what?! Thank God
you weren't killed!" The next day, they showed me the
proper crosswalks, many of which were located near fire
hydrants. Chuckling, I teased, "I'll be like a dog pissing
at every hydrant!" All kidding aside, however, these helpful markers serve as valuable reminders of crosswalks.

In April, I began volunteering at Manor Care at Summer Trace with independent living, assisted living apartments, and a long-term care facility where I had done
many things such as assisting with crafts, observing a
current events discussion on the Pacers, playing a triv-
ia game that the activities director suggested regarding

identifying famous people whose surnames began with the letter A, and assisting with Bingo by holding up large print flash cards giving Bingo numbers in front of a quadriplegic resident who called them while I wrote them down on a tally sheet as a checklist for each number called. Visiting with a resident who would not talk gave me an inspiration to sing some Big Band Era songs such as "Sentimental Journey," "Body and Soul," and "Embraceable You." To my astonishment, she sang along with me.

The remaining weeks of spring and summer, 2018, whizzed by in a whirl of many other pleasure-filled activities, such as a presentation at the library on the Bronte sisters, a strawberry festival at Crawfordsville, and a circus at Peru, Indiana, which promotes talent of aspiring circus performers. Though considered amateurs, they conducted themselves professionally.

Nancy, John, and I also toured a brand-new building housing Bosma Enterprises for the Blind. With roots reaching back to 1915, Bosma Enterprises now called "Bosma Visionary Opportunities Foundation," has decades of experience in helping Hoosiers with vision loss achieve independence. Bosma's rehabilitation program helped nearly 800 people last year; and as it plans, it is looking forward to assisting even more of Indiana's almost 160,000 people who are blind or visually impaired.

Through its rehabilitation services and job training and employment programs, Bosma teaches people experiencing vision loss how to successfully navigate their lives and jobs. Doing so, hopefully, its clients grow in their abilities and confidence—a journey that its trainers call "progressing from tears to cheers". Bosma is helping them achieve true self-sufficiency, challenge misperceptions, and break barriers. Like the Michigan Commission for the Blind Training Center for which I worked, it offers programs in personal adjustment training, job readiness, higher education readiness; but unlike the Michigan Commission for the Blind Training Center, it has expanded to community service for seniors. It produces surgical kits including plastic gloves, Skilcraft Ice Melt, warehousing, and contract packaging.

Another highlight for me was visiting Stream Cliff Herb Farm, located at 8225 South County Road in Commiskey, Indiana. Strolling along colonial-style paths immerses visitors into a pastoral paradise of quilt-shaped gardens.

Not for sighted only, the Nine-Patch Quilt-shaped herb garden and the path to the Log Cabin Garden beckoned visitors to touch and smell the catnip, lamb's ear, catmint, and scented geraniums while a fountain rippled along a rock wall and a rooster crowed in the distance.

As the shady romantic gardens invited passers-by to relax and cool off on humid summer days, tantalizing aromas of sautéed vegetables, tarragon chicken, sage pork chops, warm berry cobblers, and baked pies attract guests to the tearoom. Entering the Twigs and Sprigs Tearoom left me with the impression of vacationing in an English countryside cottage surrounded by colorful flowers, furnished with a floral mural in one room, polished hardwood floors, simple tables and chairs, and pink flowered valances matching the tablecloths which contribute to a homey atmosphere. Herbs and fresh ingredients were used to prepare a wide variety of gourmet sandwiches, entrees, salads, soups, desserts, and beverages. Edible flowers, such as pansies, nasturtiums, and rose petals, and culinary herbs alongside the blossoms garnished plates.

Stream Cliff Herb Farm, Tearoom, and Winery fascinated me for several reasons. I found that without sacrificing modern conveniences, this interesting place commemorated a riveting pioneer and Civil War history. Furthermore, visiting there did not require long, overnight stays away from home. At this farm, I could have fun in an atmosphere that created a carefree feeling alleviating the stresses of my life.

These activities helped mitigate frustration over cloudiness regarding God's ministry for me, a gnawing spiritual hunger I have experienced not yet knowing many of the parishioners at St. Louis de Montfort, and the uncertainty of belonging to any choir. Since I had sung in the Kalamazoo Community Chorale for 34 years, music, therefore, had played a vital role in my life. Here, choral singing appears to be a very remote idea, either due to mandatory sight-reading requirements, lack of consistent public transportation, or no success regarding choir members volunteering transportation to rehearsals. Sis consoled me by reassuring me that singing praises to God in the congregation means as much to Him as singing in the choir loft.

Early in September 2018, much to my surprise, God guided me to the Prime Life Follies, in which our group consisting of five women who performed at various senior citizen apartments including Rosewalk where I am staying and nursing homes around Carmel and Fishers, Indiana. We presented a fall Western-themed and later a Christmas concert featuring familiar carols and a hilarious song-and-dance duet of "All I Want for Christmas is my Two Front Teeth" in which Lori Mansell-Solinski, Follies organizer, impersonated a tooth fairy, and I, a child with blackened two front teeth and pajamas consisting of a red knit top, red-and-white polka-dot bottoms, and matching socks.

My wish to join the Follies would not have been fulfilled without Lori, my cheerleader whose personality bubbled like champagne. From a 90-pound frame, 300-pound fireballs of energy exploded. When I expressed doubt, "Oh, I'd look clumsy on stage," Lori always cheered, "Yes you can! You'll knock the socks off the audience with your singing."

She also encouraged me to be creative with props. When I made an alphabet book as a prop to "A, You're Adorable", Lori exclaimed, "How clever! How did you think of that?"

She and Ed were like the parents I still longed to have. He was as stocky and tall as she was tiny. They both provided transportation.

God led me to one Christmas 2018 parish choir which involved only one evening practice and practice before mass. After that, the same inaccessibility of transportation to rehearsals reappeared like the Grinch that stole Christmas. A friend suggested, "Before plunging into anything, ask God what ministry He thinks is appropriate for you to consider and wait for His answer. He'll open doors you may never imagine!"

Following winter break, the Follies resumed at the end of March 2019. Performing familiar music in a humorous vein and hearing the applause of the residents has contributed to my enjoyment and sense of purpose.

In the meantime, renewed interest in bowling as a pastime resurged around mid-March 2019. Not having bowled in 40 years, I certainly was rusty as indicated by my terrible scores–70s for the next several months. With practice, they improved from the 90s to 124.

But something initially insidious yet eventually full-blown troubled me during the winter of 2020. Deep in my heart I enjoyed performing in the Follies for residents at nursing homes and senior-assisted living facilities, knowing how the music brought joy in their lives. Before long, however, basking in attention from the audience, I often forgot the true Source of this musical gift as I puffed up with pride, accepting all the praise and living for the next show. In my busyness, I behaved like a rude hostess to Jesus, my Guest, rushing through morning prayers while saying the rosary as an auctioneer rattles off bids. I scurried through Bible readings without taking time to meditate on Christ's message and its application to my daily life. Was I making music an idol, replacing devotion to Jesus?

At first, I also had a difficult time deciding what to give up for Lent 2020. Oh, I might do the standard such as giving up a certain food, yet a crazy possibility of giving up Follies for a time popped into my mind. How torn I was! God's firm, insistent voice nagged at me as if in a prophecy or premonition.

If God gave me this musical talent, why would He want me to give up Follies? Thinking about pride helped me understand and consider how to change my attitude more toward a spirit of service than egotism.

His will versus mine. I had to yield if it were His will for me to forego Follies. For a while, I inwardly struggled. After fervent prayer, peace finally enveloped me regarding God's will determining my future in Follies.

No one ever anticipated a world reeling from the COVID 19 pandemic rending the fabric of complacency while claiming millions of lives and disrupting daily routines to which we had been accustomed. Soon, depending upon the severity of the outbreak, people in China, Italy, and Spain were ordered to shelter in place as were New York State, New Jersey, California. Other states in the U.S. were under various stages of quarantine depending upon the numbers of cases suffering or deaths from the COVID 19 virus. Therefore, schools, colleges, universities, barber shops and beauty salons, malls, movie theaters, fitness centers, parks, restaurants, libraries, and bowling alleys were ordered closed, though restaurants could deliver take-outs, and essential businesses such as hospitals, medical clinics, grocery stores, and public transportation remained open. Travel from the United States to European countries was restricted and vice versa. Around June, cases declined to where even businesses considered non-essential could reopen. Who would believe that cases would spike after the July 4 and Labor Day holidays and then really skyrocket during Thanksgiving, Christmas, and New Year's holidays? Who could imagine the death toll rising above the grim U.S. benchmark of 4,000 per day and continuing to soar as mutant strains of the virus flare? Would vaccinations radically flatten the curve?

Acutely missing swimming, bowling, attending mass and Bible studies, assisting with Bingo at Summer Trace, and performing in Follies at nursing homes and assistive living facilities, I wondered why God would deprive me of all these things that brought purpose in my life and me closer to Him? How long would this last, and how would the economy hold up without collapsing? Would we all walk around like hippies if hair salons were deemed nonessential? Yikes! Yet survival depended upon adaptation.

Part of this adaptation process requires physical and emotional detachment from our former lives. I'm afraid I was a slow, resistant learner until one of Father Leonard's EWTN homilies impressed upon me the importance of detachment in developing a closer relationship with Christ. For example, he described us experiencing the pandemic as soldiers in God's boot camp. Like military recruits get their hair cut, change from civilian clothes into uniforms, and receive strenuous physical conditioning, we in God's platoon receive rigorous training in detachment which can be illness, unemployment and resulting loss of social status, and potential loss of loved ones. Father Leonard further reminded his congregation that carrying our crosses as Jesus did strengthens our faith and reliance upon him.

As a visually impaired person unable to drive and coping with the challenges of COVID 19 pandemic, I thank God every day for Nancy and John taking me grocery shopping, to church, and to doctor appointments. Otherwise, I would have had to rely on Hamilton County Connect, which necessitates reserving a ride two weeks in advance or careful planning to bring home two to three weeks' groceries. Lyft and Uber allowed to operate require special phone aps instead of ordinary push-button landline or cell phones. Therefore, these two modes of transportation would not be an option until I obtain such an ap. I need to obtain a smart phone anyway to remain current.

Social distancing can be difficult for blind people who don't see floor markers standing six feet apart or plexiglass barriers in public places.

Formerly relying on taking the arm of a sighted guide, I now often resort to verbal directions from the public when needing assistance in finding unknown destinations.

Unable to see movements at a distance in exercise classes, I am frustrated by social distancing between instructor and student at Prime Life Enrichment Center.

Prevention from hugging people increases my feeling of social isolation and dehumanization.

Considering my difficulty reading certain styles of handwriting, if it were not for my sister and brother-in-law, who would read my mail? That would never get done as friends concerned with social distancing were reluctant to read mail to me.

My sister helped me order clothes online.

For delivered groceries, I would have to log into Instacart.com, locate stores within my zip code area and notify Instacart regarding groceries I need at Kroger, Meijers or Whole Foods in Carmel, Indiana, if Carmel, Indiana were in total lockdown.

Thanks to John who installed Zoom in case I needed to keep a Telemed appointment. Zoom virtual library book club meetings, online Bible study conducted by St. Louis de Montfort Catholic Church, and OASIS enrichment courses for seniors diminished my social isolation to a certain extent.

Until the coronavirus quarantine, I had never fully considered the impact of incarceration in prison or in nursing homes. Well, increasingly frustrated at being restricted from going anywhere I pleased, I began emotionally relating to a prisoner in a cell with barely enough room to move around or to a patient confined to his bed or wheelchair in a cramped nursing home bedroom. I also imagined the terror of being grabbed by burly guards and thrown into a pitch-black cell known as the "hole" for punishment. For these reasons and with the encouragement of Carol Andrejasich, the dear friend who hinted that I move to Indiana to be closer to my sister and advised me spiritually in many ways, I became drawn to the Indiana Women's Prison. Carol also told me heart-rending stories of how she became acquainted with some women prisoners through the Indiana Canine Assistance Network which uses some of the inmates as trainers for the first year and one-half for service dogs. Those ladies loved to tell their stories and wanted to make up for what they have done. Many have been abused and manipulated. Though unable to visit the inmates now, I have prayed for them and sent them inspirational letters and cards through their warden. In one letter, for instance, I indicated how we are all prisoners in a sense, many due to civil disobedience, some due to disabilities, and others due to illnesses. How many souls of prisoners I have tried to reach with God's help I will never know, but what matters is even the salvation of one soul by leading it to Christ.

In another spiritual lesson, Carol also shared with me an email defining "Magnificat". It means loving God so truly from the depths of one's heart and one's whole inner strength. He has given us so much by giving us His Divine Son, so our sacred obligation is to make use of everything God has given to us for His honor and glory. Thus, we can magnify the Lord by praying the rosary, the Chaplet, and psalms in thanksgiving for His blessings and for trials that strengthen our faith. Though unable to sing the hymns in the congregation due to the COVID scare, I can praise God as I sing the hymns I know from a hymnal given to me as a going away present before moving to Indiana while watching the EWTN Catholic masses. See, as an audience of One, the Lord is our most important audience. Spreading the Good News about our Lord, Jesus Christ, and His blessings upon my life, I am leading more souls to Him as I do while praying for the repose of faithful souls and for poor souls in Purgatory. In this way, I am imitating Mary in loving and thanking Him.

"Don't worry about tomorrow; today has enough troubles of its own." Scripture says. A planner by nature, I slowly learned to live a day at a time. Through this pandemic He has guided me to many new stimulating opportunities and inspiring people.

I hope to survive this pandemic; but if God wants to take me home, so be it! He is in charge. God willing, normalcy will return as we used to know it. Whatever our circumstances, I pray for a more loving society toward neighbor and more scientific breakthroughs. I will be vaccinated soon.

Yes, I fought an uphill battle, but God gave me a fulfilling life. As a creative God, He has abundantly blessed me including writing this book. Who would expect this from a pandemic? Thanks be to God who made it possible!

EPILOGUE: WHY *SEE?* AS A TITLE?

Wouldn't *See?* appear to be an odd title for a book about blindness? On one hand, yes, but effective on the other, because it grabs attention due to its irony. Secondly, seeing not only with my eyes but also with the heart, soul, intellect, intuition, and imagination that God gave me have richly blessed my life.

Looking back, I believe that my life often illustrated the verse from Psalm 34:9, "Taste and see the goodness of the Lord. Blessed are they who trust in him." Following fervent prayer, He guided my family and me to wonderful people who rendered possible my mainstreaming in regular classes, seeking fulfilling employment, engaging in stimulating activities, and maintaining precious friendships.

Therefore, *See?* exhibits different facets like glass pieces shift into diverse geometric shapes and designs when a kaleidoscope is turned or shaken. For example, Mother echoed throughout my childhood, "See? There's nothing to be afraid of," to instill confidence in me. "See" also means "to understand" or "to visit."

Where would the universe be without people like Louis Braille, Anne Sullivan, Helen Keller, Stevie Wonder, blind students at rehabilitation agencies who want to make something of their lives, and organizations, such as the National Federation of the Blind? Unlike the man in the Bible who hid his one talent, they all used theirs to benefit and inspire humanity.

What if society only consisted of people locked within a mindset that what they can only see with their eyes determines happiness and fulfillment? Think about it.

Blind visionaries with metaphorical picks and shovels drive home the lesson that happiness does not only depend upon our surroundings or physical perfection but also lies within our hearts.

SUGGESTED RESOURCES

Though a plethora of adaptive devices and resources for visually impaired children is more available today than it was in the 1950s and 1960s, the problem of knowing where to locate them still exists. First, you may want to check your local telephone directory under "Government Offices" or private organizations offering services to the blind in your area. With internet access, you can also type "services for the blind" or "services for blind children" followed by the name of your state as a search engine to obtain information. You may want to check if there are preschool programs available to provide non-visual training in independent living skills including orientation and mobility if the child is totally blind or does not have enough residual vision.

Examining low-vision devices featured in the LS&S Catalog filled me with mixed childlike fascination and regret, knowing how these products would have provided me with alternative tactual, olfactory, and auditory approaches to visual learning in elementary school during the 1950s and 1960s. Therefore, I would have found art, geography, and mathematics more fun using these adaptive teaching aids described below:

ART

Portable Electronic CCTV magnifiers to see art detail and color more clearly
Raised Line Coloring Books
Scented Markers to distinguish colors with different fruit scents

GEOGRAPHY/MATHEMATICS/GEOMETRY

Teachers or parents can also use Bumpers, in various shapes or colors used to mark the location of items. They can help a student distinguish one, one-half, one-quarter, and three-quarter inches on a ruler.

Jumbo Magnetic Letters and Numbers which enable children to see and to learn tactually

SENSEsational Touch Cards allow children to see, feel, and smell cards to reinforce learning. For example, a scented picture of grapes in raised lines would teach the child to identify grapes by olfactory, tactual, and visual association.

Tactile Learning Cards: Plastic cards with raised lines teach shapes, counting, and the alphabet

Tactile Maps of the World and United States with tactile outlining which would have enabled me to feel the shape of continents in conjunction with print maps

Shifting Shapes Game for young learners allowing them to move shapes along the board or line them up

Wikki Stix Tactile Learning Aids which adhere to any surface and can be shaped into basic circles, squares, letters, or continents

Besides the LS&S catalog, parents or teachers can investigate stores such as Target, teachers' supply, sewing, and craft centers for above-mentioned aids.

ADAPTATIONS

Adopted Adaptations

How I appreciated a neighbor passing on to me her large-print *Reader's Digest* books after she finished reading them and giving me a large-type crossword puzzle available from Kapps Publishing Group, Inc., www. kappapuzzles.com. Now I can subscribe to them myself from there, LS&S, or check magazine aisles at grocery stores. Self-threading needles remedied my frustration with sewing buttons and mending holes. Though I can visually identify money, folding paper currency and tactually identifying coins avoids embarrassing situations of fumbling for proper bills and change when paying cashiers in dark restaurants or cabbies at night. I have also ordered large-print check registers from LS&S, use oven mitts, a long-ring timer with large black letters, and Oxo Good Grips Swivel Peeler.

How I love the digital talking book player from the Talking Book Library, since I can listen to books by simply inserting the cartridges and pressing the Volume, Power and Play buttons.

When I moved to Indiana, I could transfer services from the Michigan Braille and Talking Book Library to the Indiana Talking Book and Braille Library without completing an application.

I use a Samsung cell phone with a screen that displays large enough numbers and don't know what I would do without it, considering the convenience of having a cell phone available to call a cab or Hamilton County Express wherever pay phones are no longer available. I am investigating a smart phone if I can get a big enough screen which will enable me to call Uber or Lyft.

I can purchase large print Bingo cards from LS&S or Amazon.com.

In addition, I devised my own adaptive strategies, such as marking a big X with different colored felt-tip pens on bottle caps of or placing brightly colored rubber bands around medicine bottles to distinguish medicines.

Though I visually identify most colors, I place dark brown, navy, and black panty hose, however, in separate drawers so as not to confuse them. Placing solid-colored paper plates on multi-colored or contrasting-colored place mats and pouring dark drinks in light-colored paper cups helps.

Other Adaptive Devices I Use

Low-vision Two-Color Cutting Board. This board is painted white on one side and black on the other for sharper contrast in slicing foods, for instance, onions on the black side and tomatoes or green pepper on the white side. From LS&S Catalog.

Man's Timex Watch with large black numbers on white dial

TimeVision Alarm Clock with black background and luminous large red numbers

Large Print Calendar from Office Depot

Medline Talking Blood Pressure Monitor
Talking Ear Thermometer from LS&S
Battery-operated Health-O-Meter Talking Scale
Prodigy Voice, a talking glucometer with no-code test strips that allows me to test my blood glucose independently. Buttons have tactile features for easy identification. It stores 450 results in memory with recorded dates and times. It tells me if I have too little blood on the strip. When I move the meter toward my fingertip to test the drop of blood, the test strip soaks the blood without me needing to measure the drop on the strip. Endorsed by the National Federation of the Blind.

Large-print simplified register for diabetics from LS&S. If I run out, I can create my own large-print record on computer as another option, given a column each for date, time, breakfast, lunch, dinner, and evening.

Large-print check and deposits register. Also inquire at banks to see if they have them.

3.5X Walters Raised Bar Magnifier which isolates a line at a time for easier reading

12X Reizen Magnifier which helps with reading prices or material in small areas such as checking a number in an address book.

Looky Portable Magnifier with battery, battery charger, and adapter. It displays enlarged representations of text, photographs, and objects. Purchased from MaxiAids in 2018. I find it helpful in reading maps, footnotes, small print in books or the phone book. The magnifier contains LED lighting. I can change the color. If a book or flyer has light letters on a black background, I can press a button converting the picture into black letters on white making the book pages or flyer easier to read. Another button puts the screen display in freeze frame if I want to note something vital.

As aids in proofreading, my HP computer has a Read Aloud feature in Microsoft Word which also highlights the words in Word documents and a Zoom button which enlarges typed Word documents on the screen.

I have taken personal enrichment and health education classes such as diabetes, glaucoma and other diseases of the eye, adjustment to blindness, business law, English composition, personal safety, and algebra at Hadley Institute for the Blind in Winnetka, Illinois.

The address is:

Hadley Institute for the Blind and Visually Impaired
700 Elm Street
Winnetka, IL 60093
info@hadley.edu or
http://www.hadley.edu

As an at-large member of the National Federation of
the Blind, I still subscribe to *The Braille Monitor* featur-
ing articles relating to all aspects of blindness, including
articles geared to parents of blind children and achieve-
ments of prominent people within the organization.
Subscriptions cost $40 a year. For further information,
or subscription please contact:
The National Federation of the Blind
National Office
200 East Wells Street at Jernigan Place
Baltimore, MD 21230-4998
Telephone: (410) 659-9314
Email address: nfb@nfb.org
Website address http://www.nfb.org

BOOKS

Birch, Beverly. *People Who Have Helped the World: Louis
Braille.* Gareth Stevens, Inc: Milwaukee, Wisconsin. 1989.
Hull, Ted. with Stahel, Paula L *The Wonder Years: My Life
and Times with Stevie Wonder.* Ted Hull: Tampa, Florida.
2000.
Keller, Helen. *Teacher Anne Sullivan Macy: A Tribute by
the Foster-child of Her Mind* with Introduction by Nella
Braddy Henney. Doubleday & Company: Garden City,
New York. 1955.
Keller, Helen. *The Story of My Life.* Dover Publications,
Inc.: Mineola, New York. 1996.
Krents, Harold. *To Race the Wind: An Autobiography by
Harold Krents.* G.K. Hall & Co.: Boston, Massachusetts.
1972.
*LS&S. 2020 Master Catalog: Serving the Needs of People
with Low Vision and Hearing Loss*
Nielsen, Kim E. *Beyond the Miracle Worker.* Beacon Press:
Boston, Massachusetts. 2009.

CPSIA information can be obtained
at www.ICGtesting.com
Printed in the USA
BVHW060730200122
626629BV00013B/1577